Acclaim for Stefanie Stahl and *The Child in You*

"Insightful ... It's easy to understand why ... it was the number one bestselling non-fiction title for five consecutive years [in Germany]." —*Booklist*

"Fascinating." —*Stylist*

"This book is a revelation. I can see why so many people all over the world have found in it a path to happiness, self-love, and fulfilling relationships."
—Marci Shimoff, #1 *New York Times* bestselling author of *Happy for No Reason* and *Chicken Soup for the Woman's Soul*

"Practical, informative, inspiring, and highly-accessible ... I highly recommend people buy this book and do the exercises provided."
—Vex King, bestselling author of *Good Vibes, Good Life*

"I adored this book! ... My life is definitely better—brighter, more enjoyable, less dominated by fear—for having read it."
—Cathy Rentzenbrink, bestselling author of *The Last Act of Love*

"A must-read for anyone who is committed to healing, happiness, and full health." —Shannon Kaiser, author of *The Self-Love Experiment* and *Joy Seeker*

"I thoroughly recommend *The Child in You*.... We should all know our inner child, and Stefanie Stahl ... explor[es] this concept with warmth and accessibility." —Julia Samuel, author of *Grief Works*

"A thousand thanks for this simplified path to discovering your inner child. I have used this therapeutic model in my practice to excellent results."
—Hilde Wiemann, certified family and relationship coach

"This book has helped countless people open their hearts to themselves again, and in doing so has truly brought a wave of love into the world."
—Eva-Maria Zurhorst, couples therapist and bestselling author

"Many of my clients have taken *The Child in You* as the impetus for further therapy or coaching and said that without it, they would never have had the drive to really take this step."
—Jasmin Schott Carvalheiro, psychologist, mindfulness trainer, and author

"Stefanie Stahl is a gift, and her book is a miracle weapon—clear, understandable, never didactic. . . . It's an absolute eye-opener!"
—Lars Amend, life coach, bestselling author, and podcast host

"*The Child in You* is kind of a 'therapy to go.' It can be used at any time, wherever you are. . . . You will be surprised how the book continues to work internally."
—Dr. Christian Bernreiter, business coach and author

"Stefanie Stahl has the unique ability to address both the mind and the heart in a way that is simple, clear, and practical."
—Vivian Dittmar, course instructor, author, and founder of the Be the Change foundation

"Like no other, Stefanie Stahl has a gift for explaining complex psychological phenomena in a vivid and catchy way."
—Jens Corssen, psychologist, business coach, and author

"Stefanie Stahl's books didn't hit a nerve for nothing: They are accessible, practical, down-to-earth, and written with a good dose of humor. Those who practice the exercises can take away effective lessons for life." —Andreas Knuf, psychotherapist and author

ABOUT THE AUTHOR

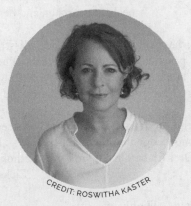

CREDIT: ROSWITHA KASTER

Stefanie Stahl is a clinical psychologist and the best-selling author of more than ten books. She has had her own psychotherapy practice in Germany for more than twenty-five years and conducts seminars about self-esteem, love, and the fear of commitment. *The Child in You* has sold close to two million copies in Germany, where it has been the #1 bestselling nonfiction book for five consecutive years, and has been translated into nearly thirty languages.

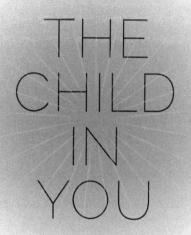

THE
CHILD
IN
YOU

The Breakthrough Method for
Bringing Out Your Authentic Self

Stefanie 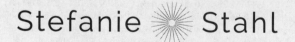 Stahl

Translated by Elisabeth Lauffer

life

For my friends

PENGUIN BOOKS

An imprint of Penguin Random House LLC

penguinrandomhouse.com

Originally published in German as *Das Kind in dir muss Heimat finden: Der Schlüssel zur Lösung (fast) aller Probleme* by Kailash Verlag, Verlagsgruppe Random House GmbH, Munich

LIBRARY OF CONGRESS CATALOGING-IN-PUBLICATION DATA

Names: Stahl, Stefanie, author.

Title: The child in you : the breakthrough method for bringing out your authentic self / Stefanie Stahl ; translated by Elisabeth Lauffer.

Other titles: Kind in dir muss Heimat finden. English

Description: New York : Penguin Books, 2020. |

Includes bibliographical references and index.

Identifiers: LCCN 2020024745 (print) | LCCN 2020024746 (ebook) |

ISBN 9780143135937 (trade paperback) | ISBN 9780525507529 (ebook)

Subjects: LCSH: Inner child. | Adulthood—Psychological aspects—Handbooks, manuals, etc. | Interpersonal relations—Psychological aspects—Handbooks, manuals, etc. | Interpersonal conflict—Psychological aspects—Handbooks, manuals, etc.

Classification: LCC BF698.35.I55 S8313 2020 (print) |

LCC BF698.35.I55 (ebook) | DDC 158—dc23

LC record available at https://lccn.loc.gov/2020024745

LC ebook record available at https://lccn.loc.gov/2020024746

Printed in the United States of America

4th Printing

Book design by Daniel Lagin

Contents

Meditations available for download:
    For more intensive work with your inner child, Stefanie Stahl recorded two imaginary journeys: *The Shadow Child Meditation* and *The Sun Child Meditation*. You can download them for free at stefaniestahl.com.

Most of the shadows of this life are caused by standing in one's own sunshine.

—RALPH WALDO EMERSON

The Child in You

The Child in You Wants
to Find a Home

Everybody needs a place where they feel protected, secure, and welcome. Everybody yearns for a place where they can relax and be fully themselves. Ideally, the childhood home was one such place. For those of us who felt accepted and loved by our parents, our home provided this warmth. It was a heartwarming place—the very thing that everybody yearns for. And we internalize this feeling from childhood—that of being accepted and welcome—as a fundamental, positive attitude toward life that accompanies us through adulthood: we feel secure in the world and in our own life. We're self-confident and trusting of others. There's the notion of basic trust, which is like a home within ourselves, providing us with internal support and protection.

Many people, however, associate their childhood with

largely negative experiences, some even traumatic. Others had an unhappy childhood, but have repressed those memories. They can barely recall what happened. Then there are those who believe their childhood was "normal" or even "happy," only to discover, upon closer examination, that they have been deluding themselves. And though people may attempt to repress or, as an adult, downplay childhood experiences of insecurity or rejection, there are moments in everyday life that will reveal how underdeveloped their basic trust remains. They have self-esteem issues and frequently doubt that they are welcome and that their coworkers, romantic partner, boss, or new friend truly likes them. They don't really like themselves all that much, they have a range of insecurities, and they often struggle in relationships. Unable to develop basic trust, they therefore lack a sense of internal support. Instead, they hope that others will provide them with these feelings of security, protection, stability, and home. They search for home with their partner, their colleagues, in their softball league, or online, only to be disappointed: other people can provide this feeling of home sporadically at best. Those who lack a home on the inside will never find one on the outside. They can't tell that they're caught in a trap.

When we talk about these childhood influences—which, along with our genetic makeup, largely define our character and self-esteem—we are discussing a part of our personality referred to in psychology as the "inner child." In other words, the inner child represents the sum of impressions made on us as children—the good and the bad, experienced through our parents and other important figures. We don't consciously remember most of these experiences. They are, however, permanently etched on our unconscious mind. It's safe to say that the inner child is a significant part of the unconscious. It's the fears, concerns, and adversities we have experienced from the cradle onward. On the other hand, it also represents all the positive influences from our youth.

The negative influences are what primarily plague us as adults. After all, the child within us works hard not to relive the humiliations and injuries it suffered during childhood. At the same time, this child still yearns for the feelings of security and approval that came up short back then. These fears and desires are active in the recesses of our consciousness. On the conscious level, we are independent adults living our lives. On the unconscious level, however, our inner child exercises significant sway over our perception, behavior, and ways of feeling and thinking. It's far stronger than our intellect, in fact. It has been scientifically proven that the unconscious is an incredibly powerful mental force that steers upward of 80 to 90 percent of our experiences and actions.

An example to illustrate: Michael loses his temper every time his partner, Sarah, forgets something that's important to him. She recently forgot to buy his favorite kind of chips while grocery shopping, and he completely flipped out. Sarah was stunned—to her, it was just a bag of chips. To Michael, mean-while, it was as if the world were ending. What was going on?

Michael doesn't realize that it's his inner child that feels disregarded and disrespected when Sarah forgets something important to him, even if that's just a bag of chips. He doesn't know that the reason for his rage isn't Sarah and the forgotten snack, but rather a deep wound from the past: namely the fact that his mother did not take his wishes seriously when he was a child. With her shopping mistake, Sarah unwittingly poured salt in this old wound. Since Michael doesn't see the connection between his reaction toward Sarah and his experiences with his mother, however, his own influence over his feelings and behavior is limited. The fight about chips isn't an isolated event. Michael and Sarah fight frequently about mundane things, because neither is aware of what their disagreements are *truly* about, and because—like Michael—Sarah is governed by her inner child. Her inner child is sensitive to criticism, be-cause when she was young, she could rarely do anything right for her parents. As a result, Michael's outbursts trigger old child-hood feelings in Sarah, making her feel small and worthless, irritated and offended. Sometimes Michael and Sarah even think it would be better to split up, because they bicker so frequently and hurt each other so deeply.

If each were attuned to what their inner child desired and the pain it felt, though, Michael and Sarah could share these insights rather than fighting superficially about a forgotten bag of chips or an overly critical remark. They would certainly get along much better, growing closer instead of attacking one another.

That said, ignorance of the inner child doesn't cause conflict only in romantic relationships. Whenever we're aware of the backstory, it's plain that most disagreements aren't two self-possessed adults collaborating to solve a problem; instead, it's two inner children duking it out. For example, when an employee responds to the boss's criticism by quitting. Or when one government reacts with military force to another state's border violation. Ignorance of the inner child causes many people great unhappiness with themselves and their lives, and allows interpersonal conflicts to arise and often escalate uncontrollably.

This is not to say that people who had a happy childhood and gained basic trust are just strolling through life without a care or problem in the world. Their inner child has also sustained certain injuries, because there is no such thing as perfect parents or a perfect childhood. In addition to the positive influences gained from their parents, these people have also inherited difficult traits that can cause problems later in life. These issues may not be as obvious as Michael's outbursts. Perhaps they struggle to trust people outside the family, or dislike making big decisions. Maybe they would rather play it safe than go out on a limb. Whatever the case may be, negative influences from childhood limit us, hindering both our personal development and our relationships.

Ultimately, this applies to most people: only once we have met and befriended our inner child will we come to recognize the deep desires and scars we carry within ourselves. Only then can we accept this part of our soul, and even begin to heal to a certain degree. As a result, our self-esteem can grow, and the child within us will finally find a home. This is the prerequisite for forming friendlier, happier, and more tranquil relationships. It is also the prerequisite for leaving relationships that are bad for us or even make us sick.

This book aims to help you meet your inner child and become friends with it. It will help you shed the old patterns that always lead to dead ends and hard times. It will show you how to acquire helpful new attitudes and behaviors instead, which you can then use to build a much happier life and relationships.

Models of Our Personality

On the surface of our consciousness, our problems often appear complicated and difficult to solve. It can also be hard for us to understand other people's behaviors and feelings. We lack the proper perspective, whether on ourselves or others. The human psyche, however, isn't actually that complicated a structure. Simply stated, it is possible to divide the psyche into various parts: there are the childish parts and the adult parts, the conscious levels and the unconscious levels. When you become familiar with this personality structure, it becomes possible to work with it and solve many of the issues that once appeared insurmountable. In this book, I intend to explain how this is done.

As I wrote earlier, the inner child is a metaphor for the unconscious parts of our personality that were defined in our childhood. Our emotional life is attributed to the inner child: our fear, pain, grief, and anger, but also our joy, happiness, and love. Parts of the inner child are thus positive and happy, together with those parts that are negative and sad. We aim to become better acquainted and work with both in this book.

Then there's the adult-self, which can also be called the "inner adult." This mental entity encompasses our rational and reasonable mind—in other words, our thinking. Operating as our adult-self, we may assume responsibility, plan, act in anticipation of eventualities, recognize and understand connections, weigh risks, and also regulate the child-self, or inner child. The adult-self behaves consciously and intentionally.

As it happens, Sigmund Freud was the first to divide the personality into different parts. What is referred to in modern psychology as the inner child or child-self, Freud termed the "id." Freud named the adult-self the "ego." He went on to describe the "super-ego," which serves as a sort of moral entity within us and is known in modern psychology as the parental-self or inner critic. When our inner critic is active, we might say to ourselves, "Don't be so stupid! You're worthless and can't do anything right. There's no *way* you can pull this off."

Modern therapy approaches, such as schema therapy, divide the three main selves—child, adult, and parent—into further submodes, such as the hurt, happy, or angry inner child, or the punitive or sympathetic inner parent. Famous German psychologist Friedemann Schulz von Thun (1944–) has gone so far as to coin the term "inner team" to describe the wide range of subpersonalities found within any given person.

I, on the other hand, would like to keep things as simple and pragmatic as possible. Things quickly become unwieldy and stressful when attempting to manage too many inner modes at once. I will therefore limit myself in this book to the happy inner child, the hurt inner child, and the inner adult. In my experience, these three modes are more than sufficient for solving our problems. I am, however, replacing the terms "happy inner child" and "hurt inner child" with "sun child" and "shadow child," which are much catchier and nicer-sounding.

The sun child and the shadow child are both expressions of the part of our personality referred to as the inner child, which stands for our unconscious. Strictly speaking, only *one* unconscious—that is, *one* inner child—exists. What's more, it isn't always an unconscious feeling. As soon as we start working with the inner child, the feeling becomes conscious. On the other hand, the sun child and the shadow child also represent different states of consciousness. This differentiation is largely pragmatic rather than scientific. In my many years working as a psychotherapist, I have developed a system for solving problems that draws upon the metaphors of the sun child and the shadow child, and that you can use to resolve almost any issue. The qualifier "almost" refers to those problems that lie *outside your control*. Among these are illness, the death of a loved one, war, natural disasters, violent crimes, and sexual abuse. It's worth noting, however, that a person's personality will inform their ability to overcome these awful twists of fate. Those who were already at odds with their shadow child will naturally struggle more than those with a sun child's disposition. In this sense, people whose main problem stems from a tragic incident also have something to gain from this book. Those who will profit most, however, are people whose problems are "home-made." These problems are found largely within the realm of personal responsibility and include relationship issues, depressed moods, stress, fear of the future, apathy, panic attacks, compulsive behaviors, and so on. These are the problems, after all, that can ultimately be traced back to the impact of our shadow child—or, in other words, back to our sense of self-worth.

The Shadow Child
and the Sun Child

How we feel and the feelings we are able to perceive (or rather, those that come up short) all hinge on our innate temperament and childhood experiences. Our unconscious *beliefs* play an important role here. In psychology, a belief is a deeply held conviction that expresses an attitude toward ourselves or our interpersonal relationships. Many beliefs emerge from interactions between the child and its caretakers in the first years of the child's life. For instance, an inner belief could be "I'm okay" or "I'm not okay." Over the course of our childhood and throughout our life, we will internalize both positive and negative beliefs. Positive beliefs such as "I'm okay" developed in situations in which we felt accepted and loved by the people we were closest to. They strengthen us. Negative beliefs such as "I'm not okay," on the other hand, grew out of situations in which we felt out of place and re-jected. They weaken us.

The *shadow child* encompasses our negative beliefs and the associated oppressive feelings of grief, fear, helplessness, or anger. These give rise to defense mechanisms, or self-protection strategies, which we develop to deal with these feelings—or better yet, to avoid feeling them at all. Common self-protection strategies include withdrawal, keeping the peace, perfection-ism, aggression and attack, or vying for power or control. I'll be going into much greater detail about beliefs, feelings, and self-protection strategies. At this point, all you need to understand is that the shadow child stands for that part of our self-esteem that is injured and unstable.

The *sun child*, on the other hand, embodies our positive in-fluences and feelings. It epitomizes the happy child in its spon-taneity, adventurousness, curiosity, abandon, vitality, drive, and zest for life. The sun child is a metaphor for the part of our self-esteem that remains intact. Even people carrying a lot of childhood baggage have healthy parts of their personality and experience situations in which they don't overreact. They also feel happy, curious, and playful at times—that is to say, times when the sun child is present. Nevertheless, the sun child ap-pears far too seldom in people who had a dark childhood. In this book, we will therefore work especially hard at encourag-ing the sun child, while comforting the shadow child so that it can relax, knowing it has been seen and allowing it to make room for its sunny counterpart.

It should be quite clear at this point that it's the shadow child part of our psyche that always causes us problems, especially when we are unaware of it and have therefore never reflected on it. I would like to illustrate this point by returning to Michael and Sarah. When Michael views his behavior through the eyes of his adult-self, it's clear to him that he frequently overreacts. He has often tried to manage his temper. Sometimes he even succeeds—but usually not. Michael's success is limited because his inner adult—his conscious, thinking mind— isn't aware of the scars his shadow child bears. The inner adult therefore has no influence over the shadow child. His conscious, thinking, reasonable mind has no control over his feelings or his behavior, both of which are governed by the shadow child.

If Michael wanted to manage his temper successfully, he would have to gain awareness of the connection between Sarah's behavior and the childhood wounds inflicted upon him by his mother. He would have to reflect upon the fact that his shadow child has a lifelong wound that always flares up when the shadow child feels his wishes aren't being respected. Whenever this happens, his inner adult could console the inner child by saying something along the lines of, "Now, listen, just because Sarah forgot your favorite chips doesn't mean she doesn't love you or take your wishes seriously. Sarah isn't Mom. And just like you, Sarah isn't perfect. That means she might forget things sometimes, and she's allowed to, even when the thing she forgets just happens to be the chips you like!" By separating his shadow child from the adult part of himself, Michael would not have seen the forgotten chips as a sign that Sarah didn't love or respect him. Instead, he would have seen the incident for the honest mistake that it was. By making this small correction to his perception, he wouldn't have gotten angry in the first place. If Michael truly wishes to get his anger under control, he'll have to direct his attention to his shadow child and its scars. And he must learn to shift consciously into the mode of the benevolent, calm adult-self, which will react in a measured and loving way to the shadow child's impulses instead of subjecting Sarah to its temper tantrums.

How Our Inner
Child Develops

The sun child and the shadow child parts of our personality are primarily, if not exclusively, influenced by our first six years of life. The first years of life are so important in human development because during this period, the brain structure, with its neuronal networks and pathways, takes form. The experiences we have with our caretakers during this developmental phase therefore make a lasting imprint on our minds. The way Mommy and Daddy treat us becomes the blueprint for every relationship in our lives. Our connection to our parents teaches us how to regard ourselves and our interpersonal relationships. Our self-esteem emerges in these first years, accompanied by our sense of trust or, in less fortunate cases, our mistrust of other people and relationships.

It's important not to view these things in black and white,

though. After all, there isn't any parent-child relationship that is all good or all bad. Even if we had a good childhood, part of us still carries scars from that time. This can be traced back to the very nature of childhood: we enter the world small, naked, and utterly defenseless. It is a matter of survival that an infant find a caretaker; otherwise, the baby will die. For a long time following birth, we are wholly subordinate and dependent on others. It's why each of us has a shadow child that feels inferior and small and thinks it isn't okay. Besides, not even the most loving parents can fulfill all the child's wishes. They need to draw boundaries and impose rules, especially during the second year of life, at which point the infant has become a toddler and begun to walk. The child is constantly reprimanded: *don't break your toy, don't touch that vase, don't play with your food, just try to go potty, be careful!* and so on. In other words, the child regularly gets the sense that they're doing something wrong, something "not okay."

Beside these feelings of inferiority, however, most people also exhibit inner states in which they feel "okay" and valuable. After all, childhood wasn't all bad, but also had good aspects, such as affection, security, play, fun, and joy. It's why we exhibit the part of ourselves called the sun child.

The situation for the (real) child becomes difficult when their parents are inherently ill-equipped to raise and provide for a child and resort to verbal or physical abuse, or neglect.

Small children are unable to judge whether their parents' behavior is good or bad. From a child's perspective, their parents are big and infallible. If Daddy yells at or even strikes his child, the little one won't think, "Daddy is unable to manage his aggression and needs to undergo psychotherapy." Instead, she associates the beating with her own "badness." Before the child has acquired language, she cannot yet even think of herself as being bad, but she senses that she is being punished, and therefore must be bad, or at least wrong.

Generally speaking, the feelings we experience in the first two years of life show us whether we are fundamentally welcome here or not. Caring for infants and toddlers is largely physical: feeding, bathing, swaddling—and, importantly, caressing. Children learn whether they are welcome in this world through the caresses, loving looks, and vocal register of their caretaker. Since we are completely at the mercy of our parents' behaviors in these first two years, it is also during this time that basic trust—or basic mistrust, as the case may be—develops. The qualifier "basic" indicates that this is a profound, existential experience. These experiences create a deep imprint on body memory. In the depths of their consciousness, people who have developed basic trust also have trust in themselves, the fundamental prerequisite for trusting others. Those who never attained basic trust, meanwhile, feel deeply insecure and meet other people with suspicion. People who developed basic trust frequently find themselves channeling their sun child. If this trust was never acquired, however, the shadow child will come to occupy a lot of space.

Neurological studies have now shown that young children who experience a lot of toxic stress—for instance, those who are mistreated in some way—will release higher levels of stress hormones throughout their life. This makes them more susceptible to stress as adults: they respond more extremely and with greater sensitivity to stressors, and they are mentally less resilient than people whose childhoods were defined primarily by security and nurturing. Expressed in terms of our imagery, this first group of people largely identifies with their shadow child.

The other formative years are also very important and influential, of course. People other than our parents help shape us, too, such as grandparents, fellow students, or teachers. I have limited myself to the influence of parents (or primary guardians) in this book, because it would otherwise go on too long, but if your experiences with peers, a teacher, or your grandma were especially important to you, you may use them as the focus for any of the exercises in this book.

We are unable to remember the first two years of life with our conscious mind—that is, the adult-self—despite the deep imprint these years have made on our unconscious. Most people's first memories start around kindergarten age, or later. From this point in time onward, we can remember how Mommy and Daddy treated us, and what our relationship with them was like.

Side Note: A Plea
for Self-Awareness

Reflection and reflecting are a psychologist's favorite words, and with good reason: a reflective person has access to his inner motives, feelings, and thoughts, and is able to see the (psycho)logical connection between them and his actions. Because he's keeping an eye on his dark side, he's better able to keep it in check. For instance, he'll recognize that the aversion he feels toward his coworker isn't actually because she's supposedly unfriendly—it's because of the envy he feels at her success. By seeing this in himself, he will likely conclude that it really wouldn't be fair to target this person. Chances are good he'll behave amicably toward her and manage to regulate his green-eyed monster internally. Because he has access to his feelings of envy and inferiority, he also has the ability to sway these feelings in a more positive direction; for instance, he may remind himself of the many accomplishments he has had in his own life, and that he has reason to be thankful. Were he unable to admit that his coworker's success rubbed his ego the wrong way, he may have felt tempted to attack her, if only with a few verbal jabs to cut her down—even in front of others.

This brief example illustrates that it isn't just about finding a solution to our own problems. It's also about behaving in a socially acceptable way. Self-awareness and reflection are valuable, not only for the self, but for society. If left unchecked, feelings of powerlessness and inferiority in particular can cause us to compensate in socially unacceptable ways, exhibiting an excessive thirst for power and recognition. When we identify with our shadow child, it can distort our perception. From the perspective of the shadow child, the "other person" is always bigger than we are, and this difference in stature leads us to assume that the supposed "big guy" has evil intentions, as we've already seen with Michael and Sarah. Since Michael doesn't see the connection between his anger and his scars from early childhood, he views himself as the victim of Sarah's "ignorance and disrespect." In his eyes, she mutates into the perpetrator, and with that, the sparring begins. And in this case, it's just lovers quarreling. In other, far more serious circumstances, it's heads of state causing destruction to entire nations, power-hungry for lack of self-reflection.

It is therefore my objective to show my readers that self-awareness is not only the best way to liberate yourself from personal problems, it is also the best way to become a better person.

What Parents Should
Keep in Mind

We have come to understand that the sun child and the shadow child are defined by the experiences we had in our closest childhood relationships. The logical conclusion, then, is that our upbringing plays an essential role in whether we identify primarily with the sun child—characterized by positive self-esteem and trust in oneself and others—or whether we instead default to the shadow child—defined by feelings of insecurity and mistrust toward others.

There are, of course, countless parenting books that teach parents how to guide their child through each phase of early life. These guides typically address questions such as how to solve common parent-child conflicts or redirect undesirable behaviors.

From a psychological standpoint, however, raising a child comes down to much more fundamental concerns: children have a range of basic psychological needs. For example, the need for connection or the need for acknowledgment. Parents who manage to meet these basic psychological needs are ensuring that their child will grow into a person with basic trust, and therefore the ability to trust in themselves and others.

The renowned psychotherapeutic researcher Klaus Grawe studied basic psychological needs and their significance to humans. I will refer to his findings throughout this book. Examining basic psychological needs is a worthwhile approach to understanding yourself and your shadow child, because it kills two birds with one stone: First, the four basic psychological needs provide a useful system to help you understand your own childhood influences. Second, this system also helps you understand any current issues you're facing, especially since the roots of these problems can often be traced back to childhood. After all, our basic psychological needs—just like our basic physical needs—don't change over the course of our lifetime. Meaning, whenever we start to feel uneasy—or, for that matter, whenever we feel well—it's an indication that one or more of our basic psychological or physical needs are being affected. In the best-case scenario, we will feel that our basic needs are being met, filling us with a sense of well-being. Or whenever we feel uneasy, we will realize that something is missing. The four basic psychological needs are:

- the need for *connection,*
- the need for *autonomy and control,*
- the need for *pleasure* or *avoidance of displeasure,*
- the need for *bolstered self-esteem* and *acknowledgment.*

I cannot think of a single psychological problem that can't be traced back to an injury inflicted upon at least one of these basic human needs. When Michael blows up at Sarah for forgetting his chips, it's because he feels his need for boosted self-esteem and acknowledgment has been stymied. His needs for pleasure and control also haven't been met. Whenever we experience stress, concern, anger, or fear, our basic needs are at play. It usually isn't just one, but instead many, or even all, of these needs that aren't being met. For example, when we feel lovesick, our need for connection isn't being met, nor our need for control (because we have no influence over our crush) or our need for pleasure. What's more, our self-esteem has suffered a mighty blow from the rejection. Because of this all-encompassing assault on our needs, lovesickness can really get the better of us, dragging us to psychological lows.

If we view our problems within the context of the four basic psychological needs, the reasons behind them become much clearer and more manageable. Ostensibly complex problems are distilled to their essence, often yielding a solution. If Michael recognized that his need for bolstered self-esteem and acknowledgment was impeded when Sarah forgot his favorite chips, he would already be one step ahead. It would shed some light upon that dark spot between trigger (forgotten chips) and reaction (anger). He would see that he got so angry because his need for acknowledgment was neglected. This realization alone could allow him to distance himself from this psychological pattern, because it would confront him with the question of whether Sarah's forgetfulness *truly* injures his self-esteem. Presumably, the answer would be no. In light of this realization, he might respond more calmly the next time she forgot something. He would probably also start to question the actual causes for his sensitivity. These questions would lead him to the further realization that since earliest childhood, he has known the feelings of not being seen and of his needs not being acknowledged. A few memories of his mother might come to mind. He might start to see that ultimately, none of this has anything to do with Sarah, but rather with his relationship with his mother. With that, he would be one giant step ahead in getting to know himself and starting to solve his anger problem.

The Four Basic
Psychological Needs

Before I explain how Michael—or rather, you—can change old patterns, I'd like to examine the four basic psychological needs more closely. As you read, try to develop a sense of how your sun child and your shadow child have been shaped by your own basic psychological needs.

THE NEED FOR CONNECTION

The need for connection accompanies us from birth to our dying day. As previously mentioned, an infant cannot survive without it. Small children will die if denied physical contact. Beyond the realm of physical care, the need for connection, belonging, and community are also among our basic emotional needs. The need for connection plays a role in countless situations, not only in romantic or family relationships. For example, our need for connection can be fulfilled when we meet up with friends, chat online, take a coffee break with our coworkers, attend a public event, or write a letter.

Parents can hinder a child's need for connection by means of *neglect, rejection*, and/or *abuse*. Neglect occupies a broad spectrum, of course. In less serious cases, children may feel neglected because their parents, who are actually very loving, are stressed and overwhelmed by external circumstances. For instance, a couple may have four children and very little money, and while they work to support their children as an act of love, the children perceive the time their parents spend away from home as neglect. In serious cases, meanwhile, children may be emotionally and/or physically abused by their parents or guardians.

When a child's need for connection is unfulfilled, it can have a range of effects on psychological development. Of course, the level of neglect experienced in childhood plays a role, as does the child's emotional disposition. The interplay of these factors determines whether the neglect leads to slightly damaged self-esteem or to an extreme emotional disorder. In most cases, the child's ability to form connections is impaired. As an adult, this person will either avoid (or habitually destroy) relationships, or develop clingy behavior, depending too heavily on romantic partners and other relationships.

THE NEED FOR AUTONOMY AND SECURITY

In addition to the need for connection, children—like adults—also have a need for *autonomy*. For infants, this means that they not only want to be cuddled and fed, they also want to explore and discover their surroundings. They have an innate *urge to explore*. Children want nothing more than to do things themselves, as soon as their faculties permit. They feel very proud when they are able to accomplish something without the help of their parents. Even very young children will insist, "Let me do it!" when their parents try to help. Our entire development is designed around our becoming independent of our parents' care.

Autonomy equals control, and control equals security. When we talk about "control freaks," this describes the behavior of individuals concerned about their own security, because deep inside (and dictated by their shadow child), they feel insecure. The need for autonomy is associated not only with the desire for security, but the desire for *power*. From the moment of our birth onward, we endeavor to exercise a degree of influence over our surroundings, doing our best to avoid moments of helplessness or powerlessness. The ways in which we exercise influence change over the course of our development. At first, all we can do is cry for attention. Complex language and actions come later.

Children's need to develop autonomy can be thwarted by

their parents. Overly protective, controlling parents who impose too many rules and boundaries will hamper their child's emerging independence. Over the course of his development, the child will internalize the fearfulness and excessive control he observes in his caretakers. Later in life, he may impose limits upon himself because he so deeply doubts his own abilities.

Well-intentioned parents who clear their child's path of too many obstacles can have just as negative an impact on the child's development. Even as adults, these children remain dependent on others to take responsibility. Or they distance themselves radically from their upbringing and become borderline obsessed with remaining independent and free, and exercising as much power as possible.

SIDE NOTE: AUTONOMY AND DEPENDENCE IN CONFLICT

It can be hard to find equilibrium between our need for connection on the one hand and our need for autonomy on the other, but it's a challenge each of us must face. This is a basic human conflict that could best be described as the *autonomy-dependence conflict.* "Dependence" can be read here as a synonym for "connection." What's meant is the dependence a child has on parental affection and care. As mentioned, this care can only occur when at least one person establishes a connection with the child. In most cases, this would be one or both parents.

When parents meet their child's physical and emotional needs with sensitivity and love, synapses form in the child's brain that do not associate dependence with something solely negative, but also with a state of security. In this child's mind, personal connection is stored as something safe and trustworthy, and she is said to have developed a "secure attachment" with her caretaker. The opposite is an "insecure attachment," which arises when the caretaker has not proven trustworthy. In people with insecure attachments, the shadow child is marked by deeply damaged trust, whereas in people with secure attachments, the sun child has a far easier time trusting itself and others.

Ideally, parents will fulfill their child's need for connection and dependence as well as the child's need to develop freely and achieve autonomy. Children who grow up this way gain basic trust—a deep feeling of security that applies to both themselves and the reliability of interpersonal connections. Basic trust can, however, be deeply shaken in later developmental years, through experiences such as violence or other abuse. In most cases, though, it remains intact and serves as a lifelong source of strength. People with basic trust have it much easier in life than those who never attained this feeling. They often operate in sun child mode. It is possible, however, to foster the sun child later in life. Over the course of this book, I'll show how it can be done.

If children's need for connection and/or their budding autonomy is hindered, they will have difficulty trusting themselves and others. To compensate for this insecurity, they will instinctively seek solutions or, rather, self-protection strategies. This self-defense takes shape as children (unconsciously) embrace the path of autonomy or that of dependence. If the inner equilibrium is skewed in favor of autonomy, they will have an exaggerated need for freedom and independence. As a result, they—or rather, the shadow child within them—will avoid (overly) close relationships. The shadow child is convinced that other people cannot (really) be trusted. F or these people, security means safeguarding their personal autonomy. (Psycho)logically, they will struggle with forming close connections to others—that is, with trusting in romantic relationships. They fear commitment, meaning they will avoid relationships altogether, they won't allow their partner to get too close, or, after moments of intimacy, they will distance themselves.

If someone's inner equilibrium favors dependence, on the other hand, they will experience an exaggerated need for human connection. They will cling to partners and feel (or rather, their shadow child will feel) that they can't live alone. These people have a fear, however vague, that they can't really stand on their own two feet.

THE NEED FOR PLEASURE

A further basic need common to children and adults alike is the need for satisfaction or pleasure. This can come from any number of sources, from food to exercise to an entertaining movie. Pleasure and displeasure are closely tied to our emotions and constitute a significant part of our motivational system. Simply put, we constantly seek to experience pleasure and avoid displeasure to fulfill our needs however we can.

It is essential for survival that people learn to regulate their perception of pleasure and displeasure. They must acquire the ability to *tolerate the frustration* of *delayed gratification* and having their *urges denied.* Parenting largely hinges on teaching children how to appropriately manage feelings of pleasure and displeasure.

Some parents are overly rigid in limiting their children's feelings of pleasure, whereas others spoil their kids. During infancy and early childhood, a child's sense of satisfaction is inextricable from their need for connection. A baby's experiences are thus split solely between feelings of pleasure and displeasure: hunger, thirst, heat, cold, pain. The caretaker's task is to eliminate displeasure—and in turn produce pleasure—by fulfilling the infant's needs. If the caretaker fails, the baby's need for connection is left frustrated.

Even later in development, a child's need for autonomy and the experience of pleasure remain closely tied. When Mom says no candy before dinner, she is hampering her child's experience of pleasure as well as their need for autonomy.

If the needs for pleasure and autonomy are too strictly regulated in their youth, people (or rather, their shadow child) may later develop abstemious and compulsive behaviors that reflect how they were raised. Or, in an effort to distance themselves from their parents' influence, they may grow up to become undisciplined and indulgent in the pursuit of pleasure. On the other hand, if a child is spoiled, as an adult they may struggle to rein in their desires.

It's a daily challenge for most people to strike the balance between satisfying their desires and denying their urges, regardless of their inner child's inclinations. Our willpower is tested by temptations around every corner. A simple trip to the supermarket requires the honed ability to stifle our urges. And self-denial isn't the only strain on our willpower: it also has to endure displeasure. Every day, we have to do countless things we don't actually want to do. For most people, that starts with getting up in the morning and ends with brushing their teeth at night. We constantly have to manage our impulses, whether they are nudging us toward the fridge, the internet, or the bar. Discipline is one of the most important requirements for a successful life, and in these days of limitless options and other excesses, it has become increasingly strained.

I will go into greater detail on the topics of willpower and discipline—or rather, all manner of enjoyment and indulgence—in the sections "Self-Reflection Strategies Against Addiction" on page 288 and "Shake Off Your Lethargy" on page 297.

THE NEED FOR BOLSTERED SELF-ESTEEM AND ACKNOWLEDGMENT

We have an innate need for acknowledgment. This need is closely interwoven with the need for connection, because if we haven't been acknowledged by a person, a connection can never form. The feeling of connection to a person is a form of love and acknowledgment—these needs are existential. Our pursuit of acknowledgment is tied to another factor as well: in infancy, our parents' behavior tells us whether we are loved and welcome. David Schnarch, a well-known American sex therapist, describes this as *mirrored self-esteem*. In other words, our parents reflect back on us whether we are "okay." When a mother smiles at her child, it's as if the child is looking into a mirror that shows him his mother is happy he's there. We develop self-esteem through the behaviors of our guardians. Our need for acknowledgment extends into adulthood, because we are conditioned to experience our self-esteem as something mirrored back at us by others. This also applies to people who received lots of affirmation as children, not just those who went unacknowledged.

Our self-esteem, however, influences the degree to which we seek the assurances of others. People with shaky self-esteem—that is, those who often identify with their shadow child—usually require more external approval than self-assured individuals with a highly developed sun child.

Our self-esteem is the epicenter of our psyche; our mental resources draw upon this font, but when damaged, it can also feed into a host of problems. As we've learned, we ascribe feelings of instability to our shadow child, whereas we attribute stable feelings of self-worth to the sun child. Understanding how to embolden the latter and soothe the former is at the heart of this book.

All four of the basic needs can thus have either positive or negative influences on the growing child and, consequently, the shadow child and the sun child. As you read this section, you were probably thinking about your own parents' strengths and weaknesses. I will be showing you how to pinpoint the influences that shaped who you are. First, though, I would like to pass along some information to your adult-self about how childhood influences lead to our belief systems and self-protection strategies.

How Childhood
Shapes Our Behavior

W hen a child experiences too little recognition or understanding of their basic needs, they will go to great lengths to attain this recognition and understanding. Children will do almost anything to please their parents. If parents are stunted in their capacity to love and/or struggle to empathize with their child, the child will assume responsibility for the success of the relationship.

If a child's parents are super strict and expect him to be obedient and well-behaved, he will strive to meet these standards, whether to please his parents or simply to avoid punishment. In order to better adjust, the child must suppress whatever hopes and feelings he has that clash with parental expectations. For instance, this child will not learn how to deal with anger appropriately. Anger serves a purpose in our lives, namely allowing us to assert ourselves and our boundaries. When a child's parents habitually quash his attempts at self-assertion, eventually he will learn that it makes more sense to suppress his anger. The child will never learn how to manage this emotion, just as he will never learn how to assert himself appropriately. He will develop internal belief systems, such as, "I'm not allowed to defend myself," "I'm not allowed to be angry," "I need to fit in," and "I'm not allowed to have my own free will."

Later in life—typically during adolescence—this child may start to rebel against parental expectations and the pressure to adjust. Nevertheless, he will remain trapped in the vestiges of his upbringing, as restricted by his contrarian stance as he was by years of conforming. The shadow child within this teen—and later, the adult he becomes—is shaped by having been dominated by his parents. Through this lens, this person will be quick to view others as dominant or superior, and then react by either adjusting to or rebelling against them. Not until he gets to know his shadow child—which will allow him to dismantle these deep-seated influences and belief systems—will he start to feel on equal footing with the people around him.

MOM GETS ME! THE PARENTAL CAPACITY FOR EMPATHY

Parents who have little empathy for their children will have a hard time truly grasping the children's feelings and needs.

This leads kids to think, "What I'm feeling and thinking is wrong," when what they're feeling is actually right. Parents who struggle to empathize with their children have little access to their own feelings, because connection to our own feelings is the prerequisite for empathy. For instance, if a child is sad because his friend doesn't want to play with him, his mother must have access to her own feelings of sadness, or she'll be unable to empathize with her son in this situation. If she manages her own sorrow by ignoring it or casting it aside, then she'll do the same with her child's sorrow. Out of helplessness, she might make a harsh comment, telling her son not to be pathetic and that his friend was stupid, anyway. The child thus learns that it isn't okay for him to feel sad, and that he's not good at making friends. If his mother (or other caretaker) were comfortable with her own feelings of sadness, she could allow and respond to the sorrow her son was experiencing. In this case, she might say, "Oh, sweetie, I understand you're sad that Jonas doesn't want to play with you today." She would then run through possible reasons for Jonas's behavior and also discuss whether there was anything her son may have done to contribute to the situation. The child now learns how to name what he's feeling—in this case, sadness. He internalizes that he won't be dismissed, when what he needs is understanding. Finally, he learns that it's possible to solve the problem he's having.

Children learn how to differentiate and name their feelings from their parents' empathetic behavior. And because their parents have reflected that their feelings are fundamentally okay, children will also learn how to manage and regulate them in an appropriate manner.

Parental empathy is therefore recognized as the most important criterion for parenting. It can be seen as the medium by which we are positively or, as the case may be, negatively shaped.

FROM GENETICS TO CHARACTER: OTHER FACTORS INFLUENCING THE INNER CHILD

In the 1960s, a popular notion circulating in the fields of psychology and pedagogy was that of the *tabula rasa*, the child representing a "blank slate" at birth. Proponents were convinced that people's character and development could be traced back exclusively to the environment and influences they experienced in their upbringing. In light of neurobiological and genetic research in more recent years, however, this school of thought has shifted fundamentally. Today we know that genes play a critical part in determining a person's characteristics and intelligence. To illustrate, I would like to examine the genetically defined personality traits of introverts and extroverts.

These traits are expressed in distinct ways: introverts recharge their batteries by being alone, they feel drained by social situations more quickly than extroverts, and they also don't require as many of these interactions. When asked a question, they will briefly turn inward to consider before answering. Extroverts, meanwhile, are able to start speaking as they still contemplate the question. For better or worse, they will sometimes even surprise themselves with their response. They recharge their batteries in pleasant company and often dislike being alone. Overall, they require a higher input of external stimuli than introverts, in order to feel stimulated and their interest piqued. Introverts, on the other hand, react more sensitively to such stimuli and are therefore more prone to sensory overload than extroverts.

Based on the contrasting need each has for interpersonal contact, introverts and extroverts also differ in their work style, which can impact their choice of profession. Generally speaking, introverts tend to prefer quiet workplaces with little distraction, where they can immerse themselves in their work for hours or days. Extroverts thrive on contact with the outside world. They either choose careers that fulfill this need as such, or, after a phase of concentration—whether online or in real life—they require a little social interaction to recharge.

People hardwired for extroversion are more likely to feel lonely and bored when they're alone than introverts do, regardless of how they were raised and how their shadow child and sun child were shaped.

Sensitivity and capacity for fear are inherent to our genetics, though, and contribute to how our self-esteem develops. Some children are born with a more robust disposition than others. Studies show that 10 percent of children are born "invulnerable"—these children emerge more or less unscathed, their self-esteem intact, even from troubled childhoods.

The dynamic between a child's traits and that of her parents also contributes to the influence childhood will have upon her. Psychologists refer to this as *parent-child "fit."* If, for instance, a child is naturally sensitive but her mother exhibits little empathy, this mother can cause more harm to her daughter than if the child had been born with slightly thicker skin. Similarly, the parents of hyperactive and/or "problem" children will find it more difficult to respond in an emotionally and pedagogically sound manner than parents of "low-maintenance" kids.

Children who tend toward hyperactivity have a hard time regulating their excessive energy, which can rub people the wrong way. Because of this, these children often get the message from their peers and teachers that there's something wrong with them. Most will develop low self-esteem as a result, even if they have loving parents. After all, it isn't just parents, but other important people—such as peers, teachers, and grandparents—who influence a child's development.

The influences we carry with us from childhood are not solely determined by how our parents raised us; instead, they are always based on the interaction of several factors. That said, parents provide an essential cornerstone. The more unstable a child is because of his home life, the more vulnerable he is to injury at the hands of other people. A child with caring and empathetic parents, on the other hand, will be treated differently at home—if, for instance, she is being bullied by her peers—than a child whose parents have little understanding for his feelings.

THE SHADOW CHILD AND ITS BELIEF SYSTEMS

If we wish to solve the problems we face today, we must understand the substance of our *actual* problems on a deeper level. On that note, it is now important that the shadow child within us get a chance to speak, allowing us to recognize what our weak spots—our so-called *triggers*—are. Many people would prefer not to come into contact with this part of their personality. They don't want to stir up their inner pain and fears. This is a natural self-protection strategy and an understandable desire. After all, who likes feeling sad, scared, inferior, or desperate? We all prefer to avoid these feelings and focus on happiness, enjoyment, and love. For that reason, many people suppress their inner pain. In other words, they push their shadow child aside when it tries to speak. The problem here is that the shadow child behaves much like a real child: the less attention you give them, the more they clamor for it. When children's concerns are addressed, however, they will happily withdraw and go back to playing on their own for a while.

Things aren't much different with our shadow child: when the shadow child is prevented from expressing fear, shame, or anger, these feelings will simply fester in the substrates of our consciousness, where they wreak havoc without our knowing. And then we experience what so often happens to Michael: from time to time, the unpleasant, suppressed shadow child breaks free and unleashes its fury on the world.

In the professional literature and self-help books, feelings are usually all that's attributed to the part of our personality known as the "inner child." I would contend, however, that the inner child (including both its sun and shadow parts) is also shaped by internalized belief systems that are typically the precursors to feelings. As previously discussed, a belief is a deeply anchored conviction that expresses something about our self-esteem and relationships with other people. If children feel loved and accepted by their parents, they will develop beliefs such as "I am welcome," "I am loved," and "I am important," all of which strengthen the sun child. Conversely, if their parents are cold and habitually rebuff them, children may come to believe that "I'm unwelcome," "I'm a burden," or "I'm coming up short," which shapes the shadow child. While belief systems develop in childhood, they become entrenched in our unconscious, which allows them to carry over undetected into our mental life in adulthood. They have a significant impact on the way we perceive, feel, think, and behave.

I would like to call upon Michael and Sarah again to illustrate the way beliefs work. As we know, Michael's mother paid little attention to him and his wishes. Michael has two younger siblings, and his parents ran their own bakery. His mother was simply too stressed and overwhelmed to give her children the attention and time they each needed. His father couldn't compensate for this maternal deficit, because he worked all the time. Because of his parents' emotional and physical absence, Michael's needs for connection and bolstered self-esteem were often stymied. He therefore developed beliefs such as "I'm coming up short" and "I'm not important." Without his knowing, these beliefs influence his perception to this day. Whenever he feels unseen, his shadow child immediately flares up: "There it is again! I'm coming up short." These beliefs are the real reason Michael flies off the handle so quickly when Sarah (supposedly) pays too little attention to him and his wishes.

Sarah's parents, on the other hand, were very attentive, but had high standards. They set strict rules about what was acceptable. Sarah often felt she couldn't do anything right in their eyes. After all, her parents criticized her far more than they praised her. Sarah's need for acknowledgment and bolstered self-esteem was thus repeatedly injured by her parents, as was her need for autonomy and unrestricted development. Sarah's shadow child thus exhibits such beliefs as "I'm not enough" and "I have to adjust." It's easy to see how Michael's and Sarah's shadow children will interact. Michael's volatility—or rather, that of his shadow child—and his inordinate criticism of Sarah's minor failures deeply impact her shadow child, which then feels small and worthless and patronized. Sarah's shadow child responds to these feelings with anger, tears, and her own accusations. This convergence of factors allows their fights to escalate quickly.

Our beliefs could be seen as our *mental operating system*, and as simplistic as they may sound, they exercise tremendous power over us, for better or worse—that is, in our shadow child or sun child. *Belief systems are the lens through which we view reality.* That's why it's so important we address them.

THE SPOILED SHADOW CHILD

Negative belief systems don't emerge solely from deprivation, neglect, or overprotection. Parents who spoil their children and grant them too much can give them the impression that everything has to go their way—and with very little effort on their end. Rather than underestimate themselves, these children come to overestimate their own importance. It is utterly self-evident to them that they should receive whatever they want, and on the rare occasions that they don't, these kids become downright furious. Spoiled children have a low tolerance for frustration. In other words, they don't handle the frustration of their needs very well. Whereas children who experience certain hardships are better prepared to adjust, spoiled children don't develop this skill to the same degree. They never learned how to join or adjust to groups—after all, back at home with Mommy and Daddy, *they* were in charge. Their beliefs might run along the lines of "I'm very important," "I'm always welcome," "I get whatever I want," "I deserve everything," "I'm stronger than everyone else," or "I'm the greatest." This can lead to them having a hard time fitting in, and they often rub people the wrong way, whether in kindergarten, school, or later, as an adult. At a certain point, they have to learn that not everything in life is free, and that they have to put in a little effort sometimes. This realization often comes in school, where many will struggle to maintain good grades or eventually even drop out. In less extreme cases, people who were spoiled as children may feel comfortable integrating into groups and prove to be hard workers, but they still have a hard time coping with setbacks. For example, being rejected by a romantic interest can cause great distress, simply because they aren't accustomed to not getting what they want.

CRITICIZING YOUR OWN PARENTS?
NOT AS EASY AS IT SOUNDS

When we try to analyze our childhood and upbringing, many of us feel resistant to blaming our parents for our problems. My clients frequently feel conflicted when asked to view their parents critically. They love their parents and feel a lot of gratitude toward them. My clients feel guilty when asked to recall which of their parents' behaviors may have been less than favorable. They feel they're somehow betraying them. I would therefore like to stress that we're not trying to deny everything our parents have done for us and blame them for our problems in adulthood. Instead, we're looking to gain a deeper understanding of the influences that have carried over from home. This involves not only the critical parts, after all, but the positive impact our parents had on us as well. We must also bear in mind that our parents were influenced by *their* parents—like us, they are the victims of their own upbringing.

My parents, for instance, were very loving. They prepared and planned for my arrival, and most of my memories from youth are happy. My mother, however, was not one to suffer weakness in herself. She was the oldest of nine, and when she was just eleven years old, the Second World War broke out, which didn't leave a lot of room for weakness. She had to be able to function. Later on, she could be a bit helpless sometimes when I was sad, since she couldn't manage her own feelings of weakness. This laid the groundwork for some of my beliefs, such as "I must be strong" and "It's embarrassing to cry." Loving parents don't get everything right, either.

Another important question is what our parents may have modeled for us. For instance, a girl may witness her loving but rather timid mother constantly adjusting to her dominating father. By identifying with her mother, this girl may come to believe that "Women are weak," "I need to adjust," and "I'm not allowed to talk back." Or she may distinguish herself from her mother by developing beliefs such as "I have to defend myself," "I will never be subjugated," or "Men are dangerous."

The norms and values reflected in the family home also play a central role. For example, loving parents who happen to feel uneasy about sex may influence their child in such a way that later in life, he will struggle to develop a natural relationship with his own body and sexuality. Thus, even people who owe a lot to their parents will develop some problematic beliefs that hound them into adulthood.

It can be extremely difficult for some people to develop a realistic image of their parents. This often occurs when one parent manipulates their children's view of the other parent. When a mother regularly turns to her children to lambast their "horrible father," these kids will come to view their dad through the lens of their mother's opinion. After many years as an expert witness in family court, I have seen the lasting repercussions this behavior can have: for the rest of their lives, these children will have a poor or even nonexistent relationship with their father. The same naturally applies to fathers who disparage their children's mother.

There's another reason it can be hard for some people to construct a realistic picture of their parents, and this is linked to children's tendency to idealize their mom and dad. Kids are existentially programmed to trust their parents and see them as the be-all and end-all. Children have to idealize their parents;

otherwise, they'd be gripped with fear at having wound up with flawed or even malicious guardians. Some people carry this idealization with them into adulthood. This can then make it hard to arrive at a realistic image of our parents that includes both their strengths and their weaknesses. If I continue to idealize my parents as an adult, however, I'll remain unable to decouple myself from them in a healthy manner. And if I can't do that, then it will be difficult to find my own path in life. If I want to understand myself—as a prerequisite for my further personal development—then it's important that I create as honest an image of my parents and myself as possible. A realistic image does not exist in opposition to deep affection. I can love my parents and value them for who they are and were, but that doesn't mean they need to be perfect and infallible. It's like any instance of love in life: if I only love things that are perfect, then it isn't real love.

Side Note: In a Bad Mood?
It Could Be Genetic

When it comes to negative influences, a mere handful of bad experiences might be all it takes to leave deep impressions on our minds. The same unfortunately can't be said for positive experiences, because we are genetically programmed to pay more attention to bad news than to good, and to keep the former in mind for much longer. That's because it's more important to our survival to watch out for threats than for things that are just nice. For instance, a Stone Age family in the middle of a diverting game might have their fun interrupted by the unannounced arrival of a saber-toothed tiger. In that moment, in terms of mental response, it's a matter of survival for fear to immediately supplant the pleasant emotions associated with the game. The brain instantly has to switch from its happiness circuit to its fear circuit to allow the family to flee and secure a chance at survival. For early humans, it was also critical to their survival that they remember poisonous plants more readily than harmless ones. Mistakes could be—and can be—deadly. Our minds are therefore programmed to register mistakes and deficits. This unfortunately means that all too often, we can get caught up in noticing nothing *but* flaws, especially when we're operating under the influence of the shadow child. This is also the reason we remember painful experiences more clearly than happy ones. It's what allows us to revisit a humiliating situation years later and feel as embarrassed as if it had happened yesterday. Meanwhile, the happiness we feel at a pleasant event can fade relatively quickly. One truly nasty side effect of this gene is that *one* negative experience can overpower hundreds of positive moments a person has had. So the next time you're angry at a friend or acquaintance, take a moment to carefully consider all of the wonderful things you've experienced with that person before allowing yourself to give in to anger.

How Beliefs Determine Our Perception

Before I demonstrate how to identify your own beliefs, I would first like to explain how broadly these beliefs influence our lives.

Our deep-seated, unconscious beliefs serve as a filter for our *perception*, as we have seen in the case of Michael and Sarah. Our perception of a given situation will then influence our feelings, thoughts, and actions. Conversely, our thoughts and feelings also influence our perception. For instance, a person I perceive as superior can spark feelings of inferiority in me. If I'm having a good day, though, and feeling strong and successful, I may very well view the same person as equal or even inferior to me.

The more aware we become of these processes and connections, the more easily we can alter our views, our feelings, and, ultimately, our behavior. To do this, though, we have to create inner distance to our problem. As long as we continue to identify with our problem—that is, with the negative beliefs, feelings, and thoughts that constitute it—the issue will remain a deeply rooted reality from which we cannot free ourselves. I would like to use Sarah as an example to illustrate this idea: When Michael yells at her, Sarah unknowingly adopts the perception of her shadow child. In the eyes of Sarah's shadow child, Michael is big and has the power to judge and control her. Without Sarah's knowing, her shadow child projects the image of a superior, domineering father figure onto Michael. The shadow child's beliefs that "I'm not good enough" and "I need to fall into line" make it feel small and worthless. Since Sarah identifies completely with her shadow child in this situation, however, it is *she* who experiences the overwhelming sense that she *is* small and worthless. Michael's criticism throws a handful of salt into the open wound of her shaky self-esteem.

If Sarah kept in the mind-set of her adult-self or sun child, on the other hand, she would maintain equal footing with Michael. She would recognize that it was his shadow child doing the talking, and that his anger didn't actually have anything to do with her. In this case, Michael's outburst wouldn't unleash feelings of worthlessness within Sarah; she would remain calm. Michael's immature behavior might even annoy her. As long as Sarah stayed quiet and didn't give in to the fight, Michael would soon calm down. Once he did and returned to his own adult-self, he would quickly see that he had blown things entirely out of proportion, and he would also be prepared to apologize to Sarah. Were Sarah to remain calm, in other words, Michael's rage would subside within five minutes, tops.

There are probably many readers thinking: "But it's clearly Michael who's out of line, so why is Sarah the one who's supposed to change?" This is the classic question of fault that I so often encounter in my psychotherapy practice, particularly when working with couples. Partner A will demand from Partner B that B be the one to change, because it's "obviously" B's fault that Problem XY keeps happening. Sarah could also adopt this stance. However, she has no control over whether Michael will actually change his behavior. The best she can do is ask or maybe pressure him to. Whether that leads to the desired result, however, is still out of her control. *The only person we have the power to influence is ourselves.* If Sarah *actively* wants to change something about this situation, she'll have to work on her own part in it.

We Cling Fiercely
to Childhood Experiences

t's impossible to overestimate just how deeply rooted this programming is—and how rarely we recognize when we're channeling the injured parts of our shadow child. Every day I see people who, although able to reflect clearly upon the influences that have shaped their adult-self, nonetheless remain stuck in their old modus operandi. The *experience* they had as children, with their parents, simply feels more real than any thought, no matter how reasonable. I once experienced just how far this can go with one of my clients: As a child, Ms. B, now fifty-eight, was sexually abused by a neighbor. She told her mother, who refused to believe it and instead instructed her daughter to "still be polite" to the man. Ms. B was traumatized by the combination of sexual abuse and her family's willful ignorance. Her beliefs included "I've been abandoned," "No one will protect me," and "Men are dangerous." As an adult, she was downright terrified of men, which took a great toll on her personal and professional life. By the time she came to me, Ms. B had undergone ten years of psychotherapy, including trauma therapy, and had already gained control over some of her problems. Despite the many years of therapeutic work, however, her entrenched fear of men had not lessened. She wasn't making much progress on the matter with me, either. Then something astonishing happened: during one of our sessions, it suddenly became clear to Ms. B's shadow child that the situation was *over*—the perpetrator had died ages ago, she was now grown up, and not all men were rapists. I was stunned. I had assumed that she had long known these things. After all, these realizations were all concrete facts that we had often discussed and she had already processed over countless hours of therapy! As it turned out, although her inner adult had embraced this fundamental message, her shadow child was still living more than fifty years in the past. It wasn't until that day that the shadow child also came to understand that the abuse was over, and that she no longer had anything to fear. Ms. B was as good as cured after that session.

Ms. B's shadow child was living in the reality of her childhood, just as all our inner children do. This is even the case for those who acquired basic trust and experienced many positive influences in childhood—in other words, those who possess a well-developed sun child. They will therefore project their positive experiences on other people and the world around them, which usually makes life easier for them. At times, however, because of their extremely positive childhood projections, these people can be naive or even gullible. People who had happy childhoods sometimes need to learn the hard way that the world out there isn't always as good a place as back home with Mom and Dad. Since they tend to have good self-esteem and are often tapped into their sun child, they're relatively well-equipped to manage this reality check. The shadow child causes us far more problems, as it projects negativity onto itself and the world outside. It's now time we turned our focus in its direction.

The Shadow Child and Its Beliefs: The Dynamic Downer

We have now seen that our shadow child's beliefs can cause us a lot of problems. These beliefs have a big influence on our perception, which then has a big influence on our feelings, and the other way around.

When Michael and Sarah are channeling their respective shadow children and start to bicker, both are largely guided by their feelings. These feelings emerge within milliseconds in response to their beliefs, which have also colored their perception or interpretation of reality. When Sarah forgets to buy chips for Michael, his shadow child then interprets the situation as follows, based on his beliefs that "I'm coming up short" and "I'm not important": "Sarah doesn't love me enough and doesn't take my wishes seriously." This is his perception of what's occurred, and he feels immediately wounded, which escalates straight into anger, and the fight runs its course. Michael, however, is unaware of the arc from *Belief* → *Interpretation of reality* → *Feeling* → *Behavior.* His awareness is first engaged at the anger stage, while the deeper cause remains obscured. He is unaware of his beliefs, and he also doesn't realize that his anger was preceded by his feeling wounded. Herein lies the problem: Situations and interactions can immediately unleash feelings—whether anger, grief, loneliness, fear, and envy, or joy, happiness, and love—that "seize" us and steer our thoughts and behavior. This mechanism can even result in the absence of feelings, a prevailing sense of inner emptiness that arises in some situations. In particular, negative feelings such as anger, fear, grief, or envy can put great strain on ourselves and our relationships.

At this point, you might argue that some instances of anger or grief are justified and based on external circumstances rather than on the shadow child. Examples might be grief at losing a loved one or the rage we feel upon encountering injustice. This is entirely accurate, of course. Not every feeling we have can be traced back to our shadow child or our sun child. These justified feelings, however, don't tend to cause any larger issues. We're simply sad when a friend dies. There's no entanglement with other people, and we aren't bewildered by our reaction. The same can be said for the many positive feelings we have. Things make us happy, and we feel pleased. Everybody has these emotions. These feelings don't tend to cause any problems.

The feelings that do cause problems for ourselves and our relationships, however, are those that emerge from the shadow child, go unexamined, and are simply acted upon—as we saw with Michael and Sarah. And if we want to solve our problems, then we must begin at this very spot.

The Shadow Child,
the Adult, and Self-Esteem

The inner child and its beliefs constitute the emotional switchboard of our self-esteem. Deep down, beliefs such as "I am valuable" or "I'm worthless" provide our sense of whether we are welcome in this world. Ultimately, everything comes down to our emotional state, which can raise us up or weigh us down. Basic trust and basic mistrust are deep feelings that have been stored in our body memory. We aren't often aware of these feelings, but they're easily retrievable. People who never gained basic trust are quick to feel insecure and inferior. They're usually found engaging their shadow child. By contrast, people who have largely positive beliefs—those who have basic trust and reasonably intact self-esteem—also sense, deep down, that they're okay just as they are. They are usually guided by their sun child, which doesn't mean they don't have moments, or even phases, in which they experience self-doubt or insecurity—in other words, moments in which their shadow child is engaged. They overcome these phases more quickly, though, because ultimately, their sun child and its associated good feelings and beliefs are stronger than their shadow child. That is to say: their wounds usually heal after a while, whereas deeply insecure individuals are afflicted with a sort of permanent wound that flares up should even a single grain of salt find its way in.

The "thought out" part of our self-esteem is our mind—the inner adult. For instance, we know in our mind that we've accomplished a lot in life, that we have reason to be proud of ourselves, and that we really *are* okay, even if our shadow child feels diminished. When I work with clients on their self-esteem, they'll often comment along these lines: "I know that I really could be happy with myself, but I just don't feel that way deep down." Others, meanwhile, are in lockstep with their shadow child—they feel *and* think that they're inadequate. Even with the help of adult reason, they are unable to shake the shadow child's feelings. Yet another subset of clients doesn't think they have a problem with self-esteem at all. They're entrenched in rational thought, suppressing the shadow child. Michael is part of this latter category, as it happens. When asked about his self-esteem, he replies that he doesn't have any problems with it. He has suppressed his vulnerability. Sarah, on the other hand, pays a lot of attention to her actual and perceived deficiencies; she is well aware of her fragile self-esteem.

Everyone knows that thoughts and feelings can contradict each other, because it happens all the time. How often do we say, "I realize that ___, but I still can't change it." For instance, our intelligent inner adult knows very well that it's better to eat healthy foods, but when the inner child gets a sudden craving for sweets, the adult faces a losing battle. With food and other material cravings, in particular, it can be very challenging to regulate our feelings of desire and instead yield to reason and willpower—that is, to our adult-self.

Our shadow child and inner adult won't necessarily agree with each other, whether in regard to self-esteem or other concerns. Many people will find that their shadow child (with its strong feelings) often prevails and seizes control of their thoughts, feelings, and actions. The more we come to recognize the shadow child's influence, however, the better chances the inner adult has to regulate the child and take back control—or rather, deliberately turn it over to the sun child.

Discover Your Shadow Child

n the following sections, I would like to work with you on your shadow child. It should be clear by now that this is a critical step in changing those behaviors and attitudes that keep causing you trouble. In other words, it all comes down to recognizing your negative influences. Then we'll move on to your positive influences and your sun child. I am fully aware that it's asking a lot to spend the first quarter of this book encouraging you to face your shadow child and its associated feelings. After all, we could start with exercises for the sun child, reminding you of your resources and strengths, before confronting your problems. The overall concept, however, dictates that we move from shadow child to sun child, and not the other way around. By first getting to know and understand the shadow child and building upon this experience, we can foster our sun child with the goal that it will come to regulate and guide the shadow child in a loving way.

* * *

Exercise: Uncover Your Beliefs

For this exercise, you'll need a blank sheet of paper, at least 8.5 x 11 inches. An example is provided inside the front cover (shadow child); you can use it to orient yourself in what follows.

Please draw the silhouette of a child on your sheet, depending on your gender. This silhouette stands for your shadow child. To the right and left of the child's head, write "Mom" or "Dad" or "Mommy" or "Daddy," or whatever you called your parents as a child. If you weren't raised by your parents, write the names of your guardians. Simply include those people who were your main caretakers in the first six years of your life. I would encourage you to keep it simple, though, and only include those people closest to you, rather than noting your entire extended family.

1. Think of at least one experience you had as a child with one of your parents that you thought was really dumb. Maybe because you felt overlooked, hurt, or humiliated. Maybe because they weren't there for you, or because you otherwise felt that your needs or struggles weren't being acknowledged or taken seriously.

2. Now brainstorm keywords based on this concrete scenario. How did your parent behave? Examples of these negative characterizations could include: mean, cold, overwhelmed, clingy, overprotective, indifferent, weak, overly indulgent, too compliant, inconsistent, dependent on others, self-centered, unbalanced, moody, unpredictable, domineering, anxious, pretentious, arrogant, very strict, uncomprehending, not very empathetic, absent, loud, aggressive, sadistic, uneducated.

   Now do the same thing for your other parent or close caretaker (we'll get to their good qualities when working with the sun child).

3. Then consider whether you had a particular role in the family. This role could also be a sort of unspoken assignment. For instance, some children feel that their parents expect them to "make us proud." Or they sense the need to mediate between Mom and Dad. Some are responsible for being a good friend to Mom, or for making Mom and Dad happy, and so on. Think back to those specific moments in childhood that didn't make you feel very good, and consider which role or task you were assigned by your parents.

4. You can also add some of the things your parents would always say, such as "You're just like Aunt Elly," "You're full of hot air," "It's your fault I'm so unhappy," "Just wait till Dad gets home . . . ," "Look at how much better XY is at

doing . . . ," "You'll never amount to anything." Add these to the keywords for your respective caretakers.

Then, above the child's head, draw a line connecting the two parent names and write down what the more difficult aspects of their relationship were. For example: "Fought a lot," "Simply coexisted," "Mom called the shots, and Dad was weak," or "Mom and Dad got divorced."

5. Once you've written everything down, dig deep inside yourself and establish contact with your shadow child by allowing yourself to feel what your parents' behaviors stir up in you. Now it's time to determine your buried, unconscious convictions that take the form of negative beliefs. What kind of negative internal convictions did your parents' behavior produce in you as a child? The question here is not whether your parents *wanted* to produce these convictions, but rather which ones you arrived at yourself. As I wrote earlier, children are largely unable to gain critical distance to their parents' behavior. They then tie these behaviors—be they good or bad—back to themselves: If Mom tends to be loving and good-natured, this gives her child the feeling that they're loved. If Mom is often stressed and agitated, this gives her child the feeling that they're a burden. In most cases, the child feels responsible for their mother's (or both parents') moods, and their inner beliefs will emerge from this dynamic.

To help you unearth your personal beliefs, I will provide a list of possibilities. This list isn't comprehensive, of course, but should instead inspire you to discover your own beliefs. Again, we're focusing this first step on our negative beliefs. Our positive ones will come after.

It's important for beliefs to follow a certain formula, such as "I am ____" or "I'm not ____," "I can ____" or "I can't ____," or "I'm allowed to ____" or "I'm not allowed to ____." They can also express general assumptions about life, such as "Men are weak," "Relationships are dangerous," or "Fighting leads to divorce."

A statement such as "I'm sad," however, does *not* express a belief. Sadness is a feeling that can result from a belief such as "I'm worthless." Feelings like sadness, fear, and joy do not express beliefs, and the same applies to intentions, such as "I want to be perfect." Intentions are usually formulated to counter the belief behind them, such as "I'm inadequate."

What follows are several examples of beliefs, although the list is by no means complete. Instead, it should provide suggestions to help you identify your own negative beliefs. Those that jump out are usually the right ones. As you go through the list, pay close attention to your feelings: which of these beliefs trigger something in you? Some manifestations of these beliefs are things we've heard before from others, such as "You always give in so quickly" or "You're always trying to please people."

Negative beliefs that directly impact my self-esteem

I'm worthless.

I'm unwanted.

I'm unwelcome.

I'm unlovable.

I'm bad.

I'm too fat.

I'm inadequate.

I'm always to blame.

I'm so small.

I'm so dumb.

I'm not important.

I can't do anything.

I'm not allowed to feel.

I'm coming up short.

I'm a nobody.

I'm a loser.

I'm wrong.

Negative beliefs about my relationship with my caretaker

I'm a burden.

I'm responsible for your mood.

I can't trust you.

I always need to be on guard.

I need to be considerate of your feelings.

I'm inferior.

I need to look after you.

I'm stronger than you.

I'm powerless.

I'm helpless.

I'm at your mercy.

You don't love me.

You hate me.

I disappoint you.

I'm unwanted.

Negative beliefs that provide a solution (self-protection strategy) to the problem with my caretaker

I have to be nice and well-behaved.

I'm not allowed to defend myself.

I have to do everything right.

I'm not allowed to have my own free will.

I have to adjust.

I have to do it myself.

I have to be strong.

I can't show any weakness.

I have to be the best.

I have to get good grades.

I have to stay with you forever.

I have to meet your expectations.

I'm not allowed to detach.

General negative beliefs

Women are weak.

Men are bad.

The world is bad/dangerous.

Nothing comes free in life.

It's bound to fail, anyway.

Talking won't get us anywhere.

Trust is good, control is better.

Write down your beliefs in the belly of your child silhouette (see shadow child image inside the front cover).

Your negative beliefs are the reason for the problems you have in life, provided you play a part in the issue—in other words, these beliefs are at the root of every problem, except those considered twists of fate. So, whether you experience issues at work, in your relationships, or with your lifestyle, or if you suffer from anxiety, depression, or compulsions—whatever your problem, its cause can always be traced back to your negative beliefs. These beliefs are programmed to disturb you. However varied and complicated your problems may appear on the surface, upon closer inspection, you'll discover that they can all be whittled down to a simple basic structure. The objective of this book is to help you learn to recognize and change these structures.

Once you've written down all your negative beliefs (however many that may be), let's move on to the next step.

● ● ●

Exercise: Sense Your Shadow Child

In the following exercise, we will focus on deliberately feeling what your negative beliefs trigger in you. These are the feelings, after all, that can send us instantaneously and intractably into an emotional impasse. When you're channeling your shadow child, for instance, and a belief such as "There's no way

I can do this" is currently activated, the associated feelings can be crippling. The more adept we are at identifying these feelings, the better positioned we are to regulate them or ensure that they arise far less frequently.

All our feelings—be it joy, love, shame, fear, or grief—have a level of physical expression. This surely comes as no surprise to you, especially with regard to feelings of fear: you've probably felt your heart race, knees go weak, or hands start shaking when you were scared. Less intense emotions also manifest themselves physically; otherwise, you wouldn't even perceive them. In some, grief can cause heaviness in the chest and constriction of the throat. Many people experience "tingles" of joy. Every feeling thus expresses itself on a physical level, even if we don't consciously realize it, because we aren't accustomed to paying attention to these sensations. To demonstrate this fact, think of a really nice memory. A situation in which you were very happy. Dive deep into this recollection by closing your eyes and experiencing it with all of your senses—seeing, hearing, smelling, tasting, feeling. Then take note of the feelings this memory releases in your chest and belly. For instance, your chest grows warm, there's a tug in your belly, your heart starts pounding . . .

UNCOVER YOUR CORE BELIEFS

Now I'd like to ask you to take out your list of beliefs again. Please go through it line by line—it's best if you read each sentence out loud. Identify between one and three negative sentences that most resonate and bring you down. These are your so-called *core beliefs*. You can also ascertain your core beliefs by thinking about the situations that make you flip out or feel hurt, or that you're very ashamed of. Imagine if we asked Michael, from our opening example, "What makes you flip out, even if you're embarrassed as it's happening?" and "What is the deeper thought that makes you lose your cool?" He'd have a quick response: "She doesn't take me seriously!" And there we have his core belief.

Core beliefs are your most important beliefs—or most important belief, if you've discovered there's only one. Other beliefs tend to be variations on this one.

Once you have discovered this belief or beliefs, please close your eyes and turn your focus inward to the chest and belly area. What feelings do these statements release in you? We're looking for feelings that make their presence known physically, through sensations of pressure, tugging, tingling, heart palpitation, and so on.

Feelings are probably surfacing in you now that you have long known. Maybe you're even feeling that, like Michael and Sarah, you habitually end up in this emotional state, which either blocks you or leads you to snap, despair, run away, or whatever else. There's a good chance that this exercise makes you feel pretty terrible and sad, because your negative influences have been thrown into such harsh relief. Allow these feelings for a moment—they're important to the healing process. It's enough just to perceive them briefly, and then you can back out again. The idea that we have to live out all of our feelings in order to process them has been proven false. On the contrary: It isn't good to wallow in a negative emotional state for too long.

The reason I'm asking you to tap into this feeling in the first place is to help you become self-aware, which will allow you to recognize the moment you start to slip into this inner state. The sooner we are able to catch negative feelings surfacing within us, the better positioned we are to regulate them. However, if we're already boiling with rage or suffering extreme despair, it can be almost impossible to redirect these intense feelings. "Early detection" is the mother of preventive measures, whether in medicine or psychology.

Please note the feelings you had during this exercise in the belly of your child silhouette (see shadow child image inside the front cover).

HOW TO SNAP OUT OF IT

If you experience difficulty returning from this feeling, try distracting yourself with other things. Facile as it may sound, distraction is one of the most effective methods for snapping out of a negative emotional state. The brain doesn't have the capacity to do multiple things at once. When something has captivated your attention, you're unable to feel pain at the same time. Try focusing your attention entirely on your immediate vicinity. For example, count ten things nearby that are either red or blue. Or think of the name of a country for every letter in the alphabet.

You can also do physical exercises to shake off these feelings, such as hopping around and/or patting down your entire body. Our bodies and feelings are closely tied to each other. We can influence our feelings by means of our physical posture or activity. I'll be coming back to this connection repeatedly.

There's another wonderful exercise for regulating our feelings: Concentrate entirely on the physical manifestations of your feeling, such as your heart racing when you're frightened, or your chest tightening when you're sad. Then expel every image and memory associated with this feeling from your mind. Extinguish them. Blot them out. Concentrate only on the bodily sensation, and stick with it. You will see—or rather, feel—that it dissipates quite quickly. It is possible to regulate any emotion—even lovesickness—with this little exercise in perception.

There's also a chance, however, that you don't feel anything when diving into your negative beliefs. It could be that you're preoccupied or blocked at the moment. Repeat the exercise some other time. It may be necessary to repeat it several times before you feel anything. Perhaps you have a fundamentally poor connection to your feelings. I'll address this problem more closely in the section after next.

* * *

Exercise: The "Feelings" Bridge

The "feelings" bridge or "affect bridge" (a term coined by psychologist John Watkins) is another exercise that can help us understand why feelings that belong to our past keep flaring up and wreaking havoc in the present.

1. For this exercise, please think of a situation from your adult life in which one of your core beliefs (or another important belief) is active. Choose a situation you commonly find yourself in—with minor variations of location or circumstance—and in which your negative belief feels relevant and real. For instance, a situation in which you feel dismissed, which confirms your belief that "I'm inadequate." Or a situation in which you don't feel respected, which activates your belief that "I'm a nobody."

2. Once you've settled upon a situation, use your imagination to inhabit the scene with all your senses. If it's too severe a scene to enter fully, it's okay to maintain some inner distance or simply imagine part of it. What's

important is that you allow the feeling associated with this situation to surface, and that you finally allow yourself to feel it—even if in weakened form.

3. When the feeling associated with this situation has set in—such as fear or grief—travel with this feeling further into your past, to your very earliest memories. Using this exercise, try to determine how long you've known this feeling and which situation(s) in childhood may have shaped it. Analyze the behaviors of your parents or others that may have led you to feel the way you do now.

The reason for this exercise and those above is to gain a deep understanding of your own influences and habits so that they no longer run on autopilot, as they do for Sarah and Michael. Gaining this understanding gives you the chance to regulate such tendencies within you—the more aware you are of your feelings, the more quickly you can recognize and respond to them.

SIDE NOTE: PROBLEM DODGERS AND NON-FEELERS

People who are good at accessing their feelings have a much easier time reflecting upon themselves and solving their problems than people who repress things. Not only do these people repress their feelings, they don't spend a lot of time thinking about their emotional processes, either. They don't like thinking too much about themselves or their lives—usually out of subliminal fear that too many negative feelings could emerge. They're habitually distracted from themselves, in other words. Meanwhile, there are others in this category who think about themselves quite a lot, but get stuck in theoretical notions, unable to gain access to the emotional world of the shadow child.

Whether it's in their nature or because of the way they're raised, men, in particular, tend to identify with reason and rational thought over feeling. This doesn't apply to all men, of course, and women who are out of touch with their feelings certainly exist. However, men are more likely than women to repress their feelings, especially feelings historically associated with some perceived "weakness," such as grief, helplessness, and fear. Most men are better in touch with "strong" feelings like happiness or anger. It's just like with Michael: He doesn't register the "weak" feeling of pain that he experiences in response to Sarah's forgetfulness. Instead, he only feels rage, which is a consequence of his injured self-esteem. Rage emerges whenever one of our basic physical or mental needs is frustrated.

For millennia, men have been socialized not to show any feelings of weakness. Only recently has a shift in attitudes begun: boys can be sad or scared, too, and idiotic expressions like "Boys don't cry!" are vanishing from parents' repertoires.

In addition to the way they're raised, men are also evolutionarily predisposed to turning off their feelings, which can be traced back to the division of tasks between men and women in the Stone Age. To be successful hunters, men had to learn to deflect feelings of weakness. They had to be brave. Women have always had to do this, too, but their area of responsibility in the Stone Age (and today, to some extent) was the family, where empathy is more useful than bravery. In this respect, men are born with a certain genetic disposition for viewing the world around them in concrete terms, whereas women have an easier time empathizing with others.

The tendency many men have to push aside their feelings certainly has its advantages, especially when solving tangible problems. In the interpersonal arena, however, these men's flat experience of emotions can cause issues. In my therapy sessions and workshops, I often encounter men who drift aimlessly about their interpersonal problems. After all, feelings are necessary for assessing a situation. Feelings show us how important or unimportant something is. For instance, fear warns us of danger and motivates us to avoid it. Grief lets us know when we've lost or not received something important. Shame signifies that we've broken from societal or personal norms. Happiness reveals the things we like.

When people are out of touch with their feelings, the connection to their needs will also be stunted. Many will therefore complain that they don't know what they want. I know many men who are highly intelligent in abstract thought, but who somehow struggle to get their lives on track. They fail to realize their potential professionally, and they struggle with relationship issues in their private life. Some will advance far in their career, thanks to their intellectual skills, but their love life and family fall by the wayside. They get bogged down in abstract considerations. When it comes to making an emotionally important decision or formulating personal goals, they get lost in listing the pros and cons. These men are out of touch with their feelings, which—hand in hand with their rational thinking—could actually help provide a sense of orientation. After all, decisions we can justify rationally also *feel* good. This feeling, even if subliminal, is what tips the scales when reaching a decision.

Some people are also governed by a *single* feeling that dominates their emotional foreground, be it fear, depression, or aggression. Hidden behind these "leading emotions" are usually other feelings that go unnoticed, as is the case with Michael: the feeling of anger always leads, while the actual wound remains undetected.

WHAT CAN I DO IF I DON'T FEEL VERY MUCH?

If you're someone who has trouble getting in touch with their emotions, and you didn't feel anything during the above exercises, please close your eyes and focus on your chest and belly area. At first, simply pay attention to the flow of your breath. Does your breath extend deep into your belly, or does it get caught somewhere along the way? We often unconsciously suppress our feelings by taking shallow breaths. For that reason, I'm allowing you to take a deep breath into your belly. It's best to do this lying down. Get a real sense of how that feels. If you still don't feel anything, please remain focused on your chest and belly area and home in on what "nothing" feels like. What's it like to sit with this nothingness? Pay attention to how your body perceives it. Is your belly relaxed? Is your heart calm? Your breathing deep? What does nothingness feel like? Then try to feel out whether "nothing" might be hiding "something" behind it.

Incidentally, paying better attention can help you practice feeling. Not feeling is usually a self-protection strategy people developed in childhood, so as to avoid the feelings of pain and helplessness caused by their parents. They learned to distract themselves from their feelings. Accordingly, you can also learn to direct your attention to your feelings.

It's often enough to pause periodically over the course of the day and direct your attention to the question: How do I feel right now? Be mindful of your chest and belly area and the physical sensations you perceive there. If, for instance, you feel a tingling, a pull, tightness, or pressure, direct your attention to that spot. And get a feel for the term that would best describe the emotion. Fear? Grief? Shame? Fury? Joy? Love? Relief? You can then ask these physical sensations a question: *In my life, what is making that spot feel so . . .* squeezed, tingly, rattled—whatever the physical sensation is. Direct this question at the feeling and allow the response to emerge from that very spot. In other words, you're not looking for the answer in your mind, or rather, from your adult-self. The immediate answer you receive is usually the right one, even if it initially seems absurd. It can even take the form of a memory or an image. The answer arises from your unconscious—that is, from your inner child, whether shadow or sun. This method of zeroing in on your feelings allows you to communicate directly with the inner child and derives from a specific psychological method called "focusing," developed by American philosopher and psychologist Eugene Gendlin.

You'll see that the more often you direct your attention to your internal processes, the easier it will become to perceive them. Some also find it helpful to meditate on them.

OUR PROJECTIONS ARE OUR REALITY

The main thing you have to understand is that your negative beliefs are not rooted in reality. Instead, they're based on a subjective certainty that you picked up from the mistakes—even if minor—that your parents made in raising you. You view yourself and those around you through the lens of these beliefs, yielding a distorted personal perception. This is your projection of reality, permeated with your upbringing. What we're aiming for, then, is to dismantle this adverse projection and replace it with a better, more realistic one. To do so, it is critical that you separate the shadow child from the reasonable adult within you. The two may no longer be permitted to intermingle in your perception, as they have for so long. With the power of your adult reason, you must recognize that the influence your shadow child exercises is just that. You must come to understand that had your parents approached things differently (or had you had different parents altogether), you would be shaped by a different set of influences. Your inner adult must accept that all these nasty little statements don't express anything about you and your value, but are instead *solely* a reflection of the parenting you received.

If one of your beliefs is "I'm inadequate," for instance, your adult intellect should recognize that this is nonsense, because you are adequate, even if you've made mistakes in your life. As it is, most of the mistakes we make in life are the direct result of our negative beliefs. Or if you believe that "I'm worthless," then your adult mind should see just as readily that this is ridiculous, because all humans have intrinsic worth. Besides, there must be at least one person on earth to whom you are very important.

Children are purely innocent at birth, and if their parents then transmit the notion—even unintentionally—that they're worthless, there isn't much a kid can do. It isn't their fault. I will talk about how to use strong arguments to bolster the adult-self in the section "Strengthen Your Adult-Self" on page 149.

Jens Corssen, a well-known German psychologist and life

coach, says, "You're a shining star from day one!" This is a lovely formulation, and one that I'd like to borrow. So: you are a shining star from the moment you're born, even if you sometimes behave "unfav'rably." You read that correctly: unfav'rably, with the "o" missing. This is also an idea of Corssen's. It just comes across a lot nicer and funnier than "unfavorable."

Once it's become clear to your adult-self that you are a shining star and not to blame for your parents' behavior, you must then explain this to your shadow child, so that it understands as well. Otherwise, you will remain trapped in a double reality: the child within you will continue to think that it's small and that the world out there represents Mommy and Daddy, while your inner adult will still believe that everything you think and feel is true. This is actually what happens to anyone who hasn't reflected on and resolved what's going on inside. Remember my client who had reached her late fifties by the time her shadow child finally *felt* that her abuser had been dead for years, and that she was now all grown up? The child within her—and indeed, the child within you—was stuck at an earlier developmental age. This client's shadow child, for instance, was only five years old. How old does your shadow child feel? Please believe me when I say that your shadow child is also imprisoned in its reality from years ago, which has immense influence on your thinking, feeling, and actions. It is impossible to overestimate the impact of your beliefs.

Projection is a sticky wicket as it is. We project our own

self-perception, which is essentially shaped by our beliefs, into the minds of others. If we think highly of ourselves, we believe that others should see us that way, too. If we're less than happy with ourselves, this is the judgment we project into the minds of others. Pay close attention to how often you assume that other people think (i.e., your projection into the minds of others) you're fat, ugly, dumb, boring, etc. How often does thinking this drag down your mood? Then imagine that you live on a desert island: How bad would the same problem be then? It wouldn't matter to most of us if we *were* fat, ugly, dumb, or boring—as long as there was no one else around to notice. Somehow, it typically does come back down to what we think others are thinking. We manage to tear ourselves down with our projections into the minds of others. The mechanism of mirrored self-esteem, as discussed on page 33, is at play here.

It is therefore great practice to simply look out at the world and see all there is to see, and to stop watching ourselves through the eyes of others (which really means through our own). We end up seeing a lot more, and realizing in much greater detail, just how much is going on out there.

I will introduce exercises to establish peace and friendship with your shadow child in the chapter "Heal Your Shadow Child."* Next, I would like to examine the shadow child's self-

---

* Ahead of reading that chapter, feel free to download the imaginary journey *The Shadow Child Meditation* from stefaniestahl.com and listen to it as often as possible.

protection strategies. These are the behaviors we employ (mostly unknowingly) to suppress and disempower our shadow child. It goes without saying that compared to our negative beliefs themselves, we get far more trouble than we bargained for with the self-protection strategies we put in place to deal with them.

The Shadow Child's
Self-Protection Strategies

When we firmly believe our internal influences—in other words, when we unknowingly and thus entirely channel our shadow child—we also try very hard to suppress the shadow child, or at least to behave in a way that minimizes the number of negative beliefs we can sense. We go to great lengths to prevent others from realizing how inadequate we truly feel. We develop so-called defense mechanisms, or self-protection strategies, to shield ourselves from our shadow child's negative feelings and thoughts. Many of these strategies develop in childhood, but some don't emerge until adulthood, such as the descent into addiction. It's important to understand that most of us hold on to a great number of beliefs, which for most people are the result of injury to any number of their basic psychological needs. Most people therefore have a battery of self-protection strategies at the ready. Most of these strategies manifest on the level of our behavior— in other words, they come out in the way we act.

In this section, I would like to explain the fundamental function and effect of self-protection strategies. We'll examine the most common of these strategies under the microscope in the sections that follow.

If a person secretly believes that "I'm inadequate," they will either do whatever they can (unknowingly) to invalidate this belief, or resign themselves to it and do whatever they can (unknowingly) to confirm it. A typical strategy employed to invalidate this belief (and similar beliefs that directly target self-esteem) might be *perfectionism*. In rare cases, perfectionism emerges from passionate dedication to a task, but it usually comes from a subliminal fear of failure and rejection. There are many people who secretly strive to do everything right because of their negative beliefs. Mistakes and failure trigger deep feelings of shame, because what are they, if not the miserable confirmation of their own perceived inadequacy? Others, meanwhile, simply resign themselves to their negative beliefs. As children, these people repeatedly found that there wasn't any point in trying. As adults, they repeatedly confirm for themselves that they were right. Their behaviors in love lead to failed relationships, their comportment at work to professional stagnation. For example, they might select a partner who is incompatible, or they may themselves behave so erratically that they become unbearable to be with. In the workplace, fear of failure could lead these people to procrastinate on projects and squander opportunities. The fear may be so great that they would rather perform far below their actual ability than risk failure. Others develop a self-protection strategy defined in technical terms as *narcissism*. These individuals compensate for their unstable shadow child with a self-aggrandizing demeanor intended to show themselves and others that they are the alpha. (I will go into greater detail on both narcissism and perfectionism later in the book.)

If a child is habitually stymied in their desire for autonomy and control, they may develop beliefs such as "I'm at your mercy" or "I'm powerless." To avoid feeling this way, the adult may experience a deep yearning for *power and control*, because their inner child is constantly worried about being cut down. Power-hungry people always want the upper hand, whether in conversation, the workplace, or relationships. Many also fear commitment, because their inner child conflates loving closeness with helplessness. As a result, they will either avoid romantic relationships or distance themselves from their partner after moments of intimacy. If the person's shadow child has already resigned itself, however, it will instead become attached to people it views as strong and dominant, and voluntarily occupy a subordinate role in those relationships. In other words, the shadow child replays the painful experiences it had with at least one parent. A typical example might be a woman who dates men who dominate or even abuse her, or a man who submits to his overbearing wife.

By contrast, if a person's need for connection was denied as a child—resulting in the belief that "I'm alone"—they may grow up to be *clingy* in relationships. They're anxious to maintain *peace and harmony* at all costs, for fear of endangering their closeness to other people. Or the shadow child protects against its fears of abandonment by avoiding close relationships altogether, instead ascribing to the motto "You can't lose what you never had." In this case, the shadow child learned that solitude was the safest option and allowed it to maintain control.

The belief that "I'm not allowed to enjoy things" can be tied back to the basic psychological need for pleasure (or avoidance of displeasure). People who hold this belief often protect themselves by *escaping into their work*, because they don't know what to do with free time. Some are extremely disciplined and follow downright *compulsive routines*. Others overcompensate for their childhood experiences with *excessive consumption*. These individuals lack discipline and habitually give in to their impulses.

These are just a few examples to outline the basic way self-protection strategies operate. At a higher level, these mechanisms could be categorized as *adjustment, withdrawal*, or *overcompensation*.

Our self-protection strategies and beliefs do not necessarily correlate with the basic psychological needs on a one-to-one basis, as I have rudimentarily attempted to do here. Indeed, one and the same belief, such as "I'm unimportant," can be traced back to an injury against any or all of the four basic needs—the need for connection, control, self-esteem, and pleasure. Similarly, a self-protection strategy—such as power hungriness or perfectionism—can also result from damage to various psychological needs. These mechanisms tend to overlap in many ways: perfectionism and being a "control freak" are closely related, as are "helper syndrome" and the desire to keep the peace at all times.

As we've discovered, our self-protection strategies are what actually cause most of our problems. If a person believes that "I'm unlovable," and therefore withdraws from social interaction and avoids close relationships, then the resulting loneliness is her actual problem. If, instead, she kept in touch with other people and explained how she felt, then she would no longer be isolated, but connected to others. So, it's not the negative beliefs themselves that put a strain on our interpersonal relationships and way of life, but the self-protection strategies that we employ to counteract those beliefs. *Most of the problems we have are thus the result of self-defense.*

It's very important that you cherish and honor your self-protection strategies. They were useful and appropriate in childhood. As a child, you adjusted as best you could to your parents. Or you rebelled against them—you had your reasons. And to this day, with the aid of those mechanisms, you are striving to get along with both yourself and others. These efforts deserve to be acknowledged. There's only one problem: your shadow child has not yet understood that you are both big now. It is still living in the reality of the past, when in fact, you—your shadow child *and* your adult-self—are now free, and you can look after yourselves. You're no longer dependent on Mommy and Daddy. As an adult, you possess far better means of self-protection and assertion than your self-protection strategies. I will introduce you to these means, of course, in the chapter titled "On Self-Protection and Self-Reflection Strategies." First, though, it's crucial that you recognize and understand your childhood strategies, before we honor and move them toward positive change.

Next, I'll introduce the meta-mechanisms, the umbrella categories that individual and specific self-protection strategies then fall under. For instance, if you protect yourself by gaming around the clock, thus escaping reality, you can enter this under "Flight and Withdrawal." Or if you beat around the bush when speaking with your boss, when you really should be defending your opinions, you can categorize it as "Keeping the Peace." As you read on, please be self-aware of which strategies you employ, including those that may not be explicitly mentioned.

SELF-PROTECTION STRATEGY: REPRESSING REALITY

The ability to repress unpleasant or even unbearable realities is a fundamental self-protection strategy, without which we could barely function. If I were constantly conscious of all the horrific things happening in the world, including my own vulnerability and mortality, the feelings of fear and powerlessness would likely paralyze me. To begin with, repression is a healthy and valuable form of self-defense.

When I repress something, it eludes my perception. And when I fail to perceive something, I am unable to develop any (conscious) feelings, thoughts, or actions in response. For that reason, we (psycho)logically only repress those realities that trigger such unpleasant feelings as fear, grief, or helplessness. There are few, if any, reasons we would repress something that satisfies and makes us happy (unless this reality could actually cause great conflict, such as cheating on our spouse). This is also why people who had a happy childhood can easily recall their youth, whereas those with a troubled past will often have a patchy memory of those years.

Repression could be considered the "mother of all self-protection strategies," because ultimately, any form of self-protection boils down to repressing the things we don't want to feel or acknowledge. Every other self-protection strategy—from perfectionism and being a "control freak," to "helper syndrome" or the desire to keep the peace—serves the purposes of repression.

When I repress my problems, however, I am unable to work on them. And if I repress them for too long, it can lead to an accumulation of problems that can no longer be overlooked at a certain point. The self-protection strategy of perfectionism, for instance, can lead to exhaustion or total burnout. Keep in mind that burnout is an outcome that tends to impact the sufferer and their closest circles only. Things become more fraught when an individual covets power in an effort to stifle their feelings of weakness—particularly when this individual wields great influence in society.

SELF-PROTECTION STRATEGY:
PROJECTION AND FEELING LIKE THE VICTIM

As we just discussed, repression can be considered a universal self-protection strategy that provides the basis for all the others. The same could be said for projection. *Projection* is a technical term in psychology, and it means perceiving other people through the lens of our own needs and feelings. For instance, if I feel insecure and inferior, there's a good chance I'll project strength and dominance onto other people. It's also common for us to project the experiences we had with our mother or father onto our romantic partner. If our mother was overly controlling, for example, we might feel easily controlled by our partner, because we unconsciously assume they'll be like Mom. Or if I'm actually kind of a cheapskate, I'm quick to suspect the same of others. We can also project positive feelings and wishes, though. If I had a picture-book upbringing, I might naively assume that the world is full of people who are just as good and reliable as my parents.

Repression and projection pertain to the mental function of perception. Perception, in turn, provides the basis for every other mental function, such as thinking, feeling, and taking action. Everything grows out of perception—it could be equated with our consciousness, which is why we cannot detect its distortion in the moment it occurs. At best, we can reflect upon moments of distorted perception after the fact. The scales then fall from your eyes as you realize you were utterly misreading a situation. It can be far easier to catch ourselves using other self-protection strategies, in particular those that manifest on the level of behavior or action.

We humans, in contrast to animals, are equipped with the capacity for self-reflection. However, people can be worlds apart in the extent to which they make use of this capacity. Some are constantly occupied with self-reflection and personal improvement, while others do little or nothing in this arena. People who shy away from self-awareness are often deathly afraid of confronting their shadow child. Patty's shadow child, for instance, thinks that she's bad and unlovable. This sense of inferiority is hard to bear for Patty, and she does what she can to ward it off. In so doing, however, she closes off any possibility of working through her issues. Now let's imagine Patty bumps into Julia, whom Patty perceives as better and stronger than herself. Automatically—albeit subconsciously—Patty assumes that Julia is looking down on her. She essentially perceives herself as Julia's potential victim. But Patty doesn't reflect upon this internal process, either. Instead, her shadow child and inner adult undertake a little psychological trick: They decide that Julia is untrustworthy and mean. They reject her. Patty thus projects her own feelings of inadequacy onto her seemingly stronger counterpart as presumed mean-spiritedness.

People like Patty, who will do whatever it takes to shield themselves from painful self-awareness, are highly susceptible to projecting their own unpleasant feelings onto others. They assume motives, feelings, and intentions in others—particularly if those people appear somehow superior—that actually originate from their own emotions. Feelings of guilt are often averted in this way. We don't want to admit to ourselves that we messed things up, so we project the guilt onto a scapegoat. This occurs as easily between neighbors or coworkers as it does in world politics.

Nobody is immune to distorted perception and projection. It happens to all of us, all the time. But there are people who are downright aggressive in resisting self-awareness. It's also very difficult, if not impossible, to have a constructive conversation or work through a problem with these people. Their stubborn refusal to reflect upon their own behavior leaves no room for progress. Their self-esteem is too fragile for an admission of their own guilt. I'm always shocked by how skewed and unfair seemingly normal people can be in their thinking and behavior, when they're not prepared to reflect upon their own role in a situation. This becomes especially ugly and dangerous when entire populations become the target of such projections, because the injustice and violence visited upon them are much more easily legitimized. However, if Person A has a skewed image of Person B, then B often still has the option to stay out of A's way—that is, provided B is not in some way dependent on A.

Although repression and projection are self-protection strategies that every human exhibits, and that relate to the fundamental mental function of perception, the following self-protection strategies are a bit more specific and individualized. Since they manifest in our outward behaviors, they're that much easier to recognize and change.

SELF-PROTECTION STRATEGY: PERFECTIONISM, OBSESSION WITH BEAUTY, AND YEARNING FOR RECOGNITION

Typical beliefs: "I'm inadequate," "I'm not allowed to make mistakes," "I'm bad," "I'm ugly," "I'm worthless," "I'm a loser."

People who are insecure about their self-worth usually

live their lives on the defensive. They don't want to provide any open targets. Perfect means flawless. Perfectionists run the risk of overexerting themselves—after all, from the inside, a hamster wheel looks like a career ladder. The problem with this strategy is that "enough" doesn't exist. There's always something higher, further, better. These people are in constant pursuit of their own demands. No sooner is one trophy won than the next must be acquired. Accomplishments provide only temporary relief. They primarily please the inner adult, whereas the shadow child remains unimpressed. External success does nothing to heal the shadow child's deep wounds. The shadow child remains confined to its past reality, adamant about its inadequacy. This is why many objectively successful people remain saddled with self-doubt and are never truly happy with themselves. They often attribute their success to luck and feel that they don't deserve what they have.

One form of perfectionism is an *obsession with beauty*. When working on our external appearance, we can be very targeted with our approach. Calories and pounds can be quantified, hair dyed, and products purchased. By contrast, the shadow child's buried self-doubt is difficult to grasp, making it harder to combat. This is why so many insecure people project their personal fears onto their external appearance, because there are concrete measures they can take to change their looks. Physical beauty can lead to some accomplishments, but these, too, provide only temporary relief. There's no longer-term healing.

Quite the opposite: The older the person becomes, the harder they'll struggle with this strategy.

People employing either of these strategies will try incredibly hard to gain *recognition* and approval among their fellows. They go to great lengths to be recognized, even aligning their hobbies, purchases, partners, etc., with this motive. Hobbies, possessions, and partners serve the purpose of boosting self-esteem. At the same time, no one is truly free of such ambitions. After all, we are herd animals, and as such, we depend on connection. In other words, recognition is the currency for connection and our association with the group. Intrinsic to our need for connection is a deep fear of rejection. As is so often the case, the issue is not the fact that we all enjoy being recognized and feel a bit embarrassed when we're rejected; instead, the problem is the *extent* to which we crave recognition. People who are obsessed with recognition will fundamentally alter their behaviors in its pursuit, thus losing touch with their real desires and in some cases, even with their moral values.

In praise of this strategy: Those who yearn for perfection are fighters by nature. You are strong, diligent, and disciplined. These are all powerful characteristics, which is why this strategy has helped you make it this far. You have every reason to be proud of yourself.

First aid: You have decided to protect your shadow child by not giving anyone reason to criticize you. This strategy has helped you succeed in life, but you're in danger of running yourself into the ground. Besides, this strategy will not grant you access to your shadow child. Brainstorm shorter, less stressful ways you might go about comforting your shadow child. With the help of your inner adult, come to realize that the whole success-and-recognition thing primarily plays out in your mind. You might even be nicer if you loosened up a little. Also remember that your shadow child will always demand a "stronger hit," so in the long run, you won't find your peace with this strategy. I will provide extensive details on how you can soothe your shadow child by less stressful means.

SELF-PROTECTION STRATEGY: KEEPING THE PEACE AND OVERADJUSTMENT

Typical beliefs: "I have to adjust to you," "I'm inadequate," "I'm beneath you," "I always have to be nice and well-behaved," "I'm not allowed to defend myself."

Like perfectionism, the drive to keep the peace and make everyone happy is a very common self-protection strategy. They're often simultaneously at play. Both strategies protect the shadow child's extreme fear of rejection.

People who work to keep the peace would ideally like to fulfill everyone else's expectations. They discovered in childhood that this was the best way to receive affection and acknowledgment. These "peacekeepers" learned early on that the best way to adjust to situations and other people was to suppress their own hopes and feelings. A determined mind gets in the way of conforming, after all. These people reflexively suppress powerful emotions like rage or aggression, which might otherwise bolster their free will. They shy away from antagonizing behaviors. They tend to respond to personal violations or injuries with sorrow rather than anger. People with this self-protection strategy are therefore at greater risk of depression than those who have better access to their feelings of rage. It isn't that people who balk at aggression don't experience anger; instead, these feelings transform into a kind of cold rage that often leads to passive resistance. Rather than saying what they want, for instance, they might become offended and withdraw from an interaction, stonewalling the other person. I'll examine the varieties of passive and active aggression more closely in the sections "Self-Protection Strategy: The Power Hungry" on page 107 and "The Control Freaks" on page 111.

Whether a person tends more toward adjustment or resistance has as much to do with their nature as with their childhood experiences: people with a greater need for peace tend to have a more placid, sensitive disposition, whereas children who rebel against parental expectations are usually more impulsive.

Peacekeepers often don't know what they actually want because they're so well trained in suppressing their own desires. It can be difficult for them to define personal goals and make decisions.

People who are eager to please are very friendly and nice in interpersonal exchanges, but this self-protection strategy can strain or even destroy relationships. These people are terrified of rubbing others the wrong way, and try to avoid conflict. They won't be honest about what they feel, think, or want—at least, not if they worry that this might be met with opposition. Their shadow child immediately perceives other people as bigger and better. This skewed perception can easily lead us to fall into the victim role: Fearing the person we assume is stronger than us, we willingly subjugate ourselves and do things we don't actually want to. The (supposedly) stronger person can then mutate into a perpetrator in our eyes. Our inner adult is usually unable to recognize that it is the shadow child's projections that lead to this voluntary submission. Instead, we resent the person for their assumed dominance. The more we start to feel that we're coming up short and being dominated, the more likely we are to withdraw in order to protect our personal space. The supposedly stronger person never gets the chance to intervene in this process, because that would require us to open up to them—which, because we fear confrontation and rejection, will never happen. A common psychological effect then comes into play: we, thinking we're weaker, will make the person we perceive as stronger experience exactly the thing we've been protecting ourselves against—in this case, rejection. This is known as *victim-offender reversal.*

In praise of this strategy: You make a tremendous effort to get along with other people and not to hurt anyone. This makes you kind, lovable, and a great teammate, because you often put yourself and your needs second to those of the group.

First aid: Your shadow child wants to remain as hidden as possible, making it hard for others to tell where they stand with you. Let your shadow child know that it's welcome to show its face every now and then. It's allowed to stand by its desires and needs. You won't lose appeal in doing this—you might even earn points, as you become more emotionally available and transparent to your contemporaries. They won't have to rack their brains trying to figure out what's going on in your head. Make one thing clear to yourself: It's easier for other people when you say what you want rather than withdrawing and sulking. It also helps you avoid changing (however unintendedly) from victim to offender.

SELF-PROTECTION STRATEGY: HELPER SYNDROME

Typical beliefs: "I'm worthless," "I'm inadequate," "I have to help you in order to be loved," "I'm inferior," "I'm dependent on you."

People who suffer from so-called helper syndrome protect their shadow child by offering to help other people they perceive as being in need. These people's good deeds make them feel stronger and more useful. Helper syndrome is therefore considered one of the most socially acceptable self-protection strategies. The problem is that helpers tend to attach themselves to people they can't help. They can get caught in hopeless projects, especially when the "person in need" is their partner. They tend to select partners who demonstrate clear flaws. Helpers see themselves as a knight in shining armor, riding up on a white horse to liberate their partner from misery and making them—the helper—invaluable to their loved one. Best suited to the partner role are people with emotional issues, those suffering from addiction or a physically debilitating condition, or individuals on the brink of financial ruin.

People with both feet on the ground, meanwhile, elicit feelings of inferiority in helpers, because they don't need any help. The equation helpers establish in relationships amounts to "You need me, so you're not going anywhere." The problem is that this equation rarely works out. Helpers exhaust themselves, fighting a losing battle. They refuse to admit that at the end of the day, their influence over their target is minimal. If our partner is unwilling to make any changes or accept some responsibility for their own troubles, even the most ironclad advice won't help. The dynamic of dependence is thus reversed: as the helper, we wanted our partner to depend on us, but we now depend on them, because we can neither help them nor leave them.

This dilemma is so tricky because the shadow child thinks it's our fault that our partner is the way they are. After all, our partner's problems don't affect them alone—we feel the strain on the relationship, too. Helpers are often mistreated by their partners. Our own needs for attention and affection are chronically shortchanged. Our shadow child's fears that it is worthless and bad are thus confirmed. In an effort to disprove this belief, our shadow child will keep fighting for our partner, in the unshakable hope that they will change and treat us better. In this battle, though, helpers are caught, hook, line, and sinker.

In praise of this strategy: You try very hard to help and be a good person. You should respect that. You really have helped some people, and they're grateful to you for that.

First aid: The problem with this strategy is that you tend to take on impossible projects. Try to remind your shadow child that it is adequate and valuable, even if it isn't rushing to help every single person. Let it know that there are some people you can't help. And explain to it that you—that is, your shadow child and inner adult—aren't solely responsible for your own happiness, and that other people should contribute to it as well. Of course you can continue to help other people—it's a wonderful quality. But look more closely at where your help is appropriate and where it isn't. Let your shadow child know it is using those people it wants to help as a crutch to help itself. Later in this book, I will show you how to find healthier inner stability rather than succumbing to helper syndrome.

SELF-PROTECTION STRATEGY: THE POWER HUNGRY

Typical beliefs: "I'm at your mercy," "I'm powerless," "I can't defend myself," "I'm inadequate," "I'm not allowed to make mistakes," "I can't trust anybody," "I need to keep on top of things," "I'm coming up short."

This self-protection strategy shows up in people whose shadow child is afraid of being the underdog or coming under attack. In childhood, these people often found themselves at the mercy of their parents. Like the peacekeepers we met above, the shadow child in power-hungry individuals projects superiority and dominance onto others. Rather than adjusting to those who are supposedly stronger, however, the power-hungry respond by resisting them. People who fall into this pattern want to maintain the upper hand in interpersonal scenarios. To do so, they may choose (unconsciously) between two strategies: *active resistance* or *passive resistance.* Most will opt for both. Power-hungry individuals are not the only ones who engage in active resistance and passive resistance, however. These are behaviors that all of us use (sometimes *must* use) in order to protect our personal boundaries. They play an especially important role for people with a deep need for power and control, which is why I'm focusing on them here.

A certain level of aggression is required in order to make a stand, which is why we also talk about *active aggression* and *passive aggression.* Active aggression is recognizable as such. The individual concerned insists on their right to something, argues, and attacks.

Passive aggression—or passive resistance—is not as clear at first glance. When someone behaves passive-aggressively, they don't openly share their thoughts, but will instead deny others this information by means of sabotage, whether major or minor. Ultimately, the passive-aggressive person will simply *not* do what is expected of them. For instance, commitments will be made but then "forgotten" or simply broken. Or those commitments will be fulfilled, but in a painfully slow manner.

A typical form of passive resistance is stonewalling: dodging or evading another person's advances or questions, regardless of how much they beg. The shadow child hiding behind this behavior thinks it has been forced to compromise too often in its relationship with the other person. One of my clients once moved to another city "against his will" to be with his partner, although he would rather have stayed in his hometown. He resented her for this so deeply (albeit subliminally) that he lost all interest in sex. Sexual indifference is a common expression of passive aggression in both men and women. This brief example reminds us how important it is to take responsibility for our own decisions. My client had (unknowingly) made himself the victim of his supposedly dominant partner and not reflected upon the fact that his shadow child had voluntarily submitted to his girlfriend's wishes.

Stubbornness is a character trait closely linked to passive resistance. People who are obstinate and uncompromising, simply doing their own thing, can trigger strong feelings of aggression in the people around them, because those people feel unable to exercise any influence over the willful holdout. People who are actively aggressive also infuriate their targets, of course, provided fear doesn't get in the way. Active assailants are up-front about what they're doing, at least, and thus take some responsibility for their behavior. Passive aggressors, on the other hand, hide behind the illusion of outward calm. This behavior can be so frustrating to other people that they actually appear to be the "guilty party" when they end up flailing about in helpless rage. In psychological terms, this latter category of person is known as the "identified patient." It means that everyone around thinks that the individual showing symptoms (in this case, anger and aggression) is the true "psycho," and not the passive-aggressive individual, whose subliminal manipulation prevents any possibility of having a fruitful interaction.

People who exhibit this extreme need for power are difficult to be around, because they always have to be right. Things have to happen exactly the way they want, and they will passive-aggressively forgo sensible cooperation. Here, too, victim-offender reversal occurs: The person in power, whose inner child sees itself as inferior and victimized (by its parents), projects dominance and superiority onto other people, who the inner child must protect itself against. By employing this power play, the inner child thus inflicts upon other people the same feelings of powerlessness that it is trying to avoid itself.

People who are generally quite pleasant can also experience "spasms" of power-hungriness. Their shadow child sometimes likes wielding a little power, perhaps by hurting their partner without cause. For example, a very affable client once told me that whenever her partner was in a really good, affectionate mood, she often felt the urge to cut him down with caustic remarks. She hated this behavior and couldn't immediately explain what her motive for it might be. Upon analyzing individual situations, it emerged that her injured shadow child relished the power it had over her boyfriend. In so doing, my client was unconsciously taking revenge on her domineering father.

Power-hungriness also manifests in *demanding behavior*. Highly demanding people often unconsciously believe that, "I've come up short." They quickly consider themselves outdone or outsmarted. In self-protection, their shadow child has resolved not to let anyone get the better of them. It demands that its needs be fulfilled. Power-hungry people take far more than they give, although they would beg to differ: given their underlying beliefs, they tend to see themselves as victims. When dealing with "sir" or "madam," it's easy to feel like we're just placating them by doing whatever they ask.

In somewhat more tempered form, these people are just misers. They carefully monitor their own rights, and although aware of others' rights, they're just never very generous—whether in terms of money, praise, or favors. Things are tallied up and offset. Their shadow child protects itself by "hogging" things.

In praise of this strategy: You're a strong person. You defend yourself and stand up to opponents. You are the opposite of resignation. You're assertive and have an unbelievably strong will to survive, which has protected and helped you many times.

First aid: Let your shadow child know that gone are the days of living with Mom and Dad. You—your inner adult and shadow child—are all grown up now. Of course you have the same rights as other people, and of course you're allowed to defend yourself. The problem is, you're always rolling out the big guns. The world out there isn't as bad as you think. Relax, and gain trust in yourself and others. Many of the conflicts you are trying to fix by means of power—or even those you may have instigated by these means—are unnecessary. You would actually make it a lot further with goodwill and empathy. And I'll be showing you how later in the book.

SELF-PROTECTION STRATEGY: THE CONTROL FREAKS

Typical beliefs: "I need to keep on top of things," "I'm losing myself," "I'm at your mercy," "I can't trust you," "I'm inadequate," "I'm worthless."

Another variation of the desire for power is the excessive *need for control*. Like power, control plays an important part in our general need for security. As such, we need to exercise a certain degree of control over ourselves and our surroundings in order to make it through this life more or less unscathed. Some people, however, require higher-than-average levels of certainty and security. Underlying this is the shadow child's fear of chaos and personal downfall—the fear of vulnerability. Meticulous order, perfectionism, and strict adherence to certain rules are used to stave off this fear. Similar to people striving for perfection—itself a type of need for control—"control freaks" tend to wear themselves out, especially since they have such trouble delegating, not wanting to loosen their grip.

People who crave control focus not only on optimizing themselves, but will also keep a close eye on their partner and other family members. Control freaks demand to be kept informed of their loved ones' activities, because they trust other people as little as they trust themselves. At its height, this distrust can escalate to delusional jealousy. Many a relationship has fallen apart due to one of the partners' overly controlling habits. Excessive control can also negatively impact children's development.

Control freaks are compulsively self-disciplined, in order to maintain control over their health and/or appearance. In this case, the shadow child is projecting its inner vulnerability onto the body. In extreme cases, this can take the form of hypochondria. Similar to the obsession with beauty, the body provides an object for projection that is more tangible—and thus easier to control—than the nebulous fears of destruction that lie beneath.

Another way of exercising control is *obsessive rumination*. Many people complain that they can't turn off their thoughts. These thoughts compulsively repeat the same course, over and over. Rumination can be seen as a helpless attempt at finding a solution: the mind simply doesn't shut off until the roadblock has been removed. The endless loops these thoughts run, however, are more likely to block the solution than to reveal it.

In praise of this strategy: You're incredibly disciplined and self-possessed. Discipline is a highly valuable resource for getting by in this life. You have a strong will, something you can be proud of.

First aid: The problem you face is that you often overdo things in an effort to protect your shadow child from its core fear of being attacked and injured. Your need for control often stresses you out, as it does those around you. It is especially important for you that your shadow child gain self-confidence. And a little more faith that everything will work out in the end. Try to be more joyful and calm. Team up with your inner adult to remind your shadow child that it *is* adequate, just the way it is, and doesn't always need to try so hard. Allow yourself to take regular breaks, and reward yourself for your accomplishments.

If you suffer from obsessive rumination, take half an hour each day to work on your problems in writing. Then try, with all your might, to redirect your attention to other things. Your inner adult has the assurance that, whatever happens, everything is written down and no information has gone missing.

SELF-PROTECTION STRATEGY: AGGRESSION AND ATTACK

Typical beliefs: "I am inferior," "I can't trust you," "I'm not allowed to set boundaries," "The world is evil," "I'm coming up short," "I'm not important."

As I have already mentioned, rage and aggression have always played an important part in human history, in that they allow us to protect our personal boundaries. The problem today is that our enemies are not as objectively clear as they were in the Stone Age. Projection and distorted perception can make us see enemies where there are none. People whose shadow child feels inferior to others are quick to feel subjectively attacked. For instance, they might take an objectively harmless comment entirely the wrong way and become deeply insulted. Feeling insulted can unleash tremendous (active) aggression, especially in people who don't reflexively suppress their anger (like peacekeepers).

People who are unknowingly prone to rebellious behavior respond to real or suspected attacks against them by fighting back. In this book, we won't go into extreme cases—such as the jealous husband whose bruised ego generates so much hatred that he stabs his wife—but will instead consider everyday examples, like the universally recognized "jerk."

We've all been in that situation where the person we're with unexpectedly snaps, and we're left wondering what we did or said that was so bad. As we saw with Michael, jerks exhibit a rapid stimulus-response-action pattern. They react to a suspected attack by feeling offended, which unleashes their rage, and they impulsively strike back, whether verbally or physically (although physical assault and violent verbal attacks belong to an altogether different category of behavior).

People who tend toward impulsiveness often suffer from it, too. Once the rage dissipates and they return to their adult-selves, they realize that they overreacted. The problem is that impulsive anger is very hard to tame. If someone wants to rein in their impulsiveness, the interventions must target the rage and its prevention. Prevention has to start at the injury itself and is thus one of the core objectives of this book. I'll be going into the topic of personal injury or offense in great detail later on.

In praise of this strategy: You don't take crap from anyone. You're very strong and know how to protect yourself. You're a fighter. Your impulsiveness also makes you very lively—it's never boring when you're around.

First aid: Your shadow child is easily offended. It too quickly feels it's been attacked or treated disrespectfully. Try to stay with your adult-self, thus remaining at eye level with your contemporaries and allowing you to respond in a rational, appropriate way. It can help a lot to prepare yourself for situations that could set you off. Analyze the role your shadow child—with its skewed perception—plays in this, and separate it from your inner adult. Your inner adult must keep the upper hand at all costs. To do so, it helps to have some response strategies at the ready, which I'll explain in the section "A Little Lesson in Quick-Wittedness" on page 283.

SELF-PROTECTION STRATEGY: I'LL REMAIN A CHILD

Typical beliefs: "I'm too weak," "I'm so small," "I'm dependent," "I need to adjust to others," "I can't disappoint you," "I can't do it alone," "I'm inadequate," "I can't leave you."

Some people don't want to grow up, but would rather remain a child. They lean on others in the hopes that these people will guide them through life. This might be their life partner or even their parents. The number of people who still rely on their parents isn't as small as it would seem. They lack the confidence to go their own way, and instead turn to their parents or others for approval when facing big decisions. The shadow child within them lacks the courage to determine the course of its own life. It feels dependent and small. It feels extreme guilt at the idea of breaking away from its parents or partner.

People who rely on their parents and their opinions don't necessarily have to have a good relationship with them. Some people aren't even in contact with their parents, yet they still behave according to their (internalized) rules. I recall a client I once had—I'll call him Harold—who despised his parents because he'd had a terrible childhood. He lived hundreds of miles away from them and almost never saw them. Nevertheless, his shadow child was shaped almost entirely by the values and attitudes his parents—his authoritarian father, in particular— had instilled in him. Achievement was all that mattered to his father. In his father's eyes, free time and fun were worthless. Harold's mother was afraid of her husband, and was thus unable to protect her son from his father's extreme demands and violent punishments. And although my client had already hated his father as a child, he had thoroughly adopted his obsession with success. In our first sessions, Harold wasn't even able to engage his adult-self and distance himself from this fixation. In accordance with his parental influences, Harold had advanced quickly in his career and worked constantly. He allowed himself almost no joys in life and struggled to see how such enjoyment was even possible. At the same time, he was desperate to relax and be happy, but he was terrified that if he indulged his wishes in the slightest, he might be lost to the other extreme. Some of his primary self-protection strategies were thus control and self-discipline. Harold is a textbook example of an adult who has remained a (shadow) child, even while appearing to make autonomous adult decisions and maintaining great distance from his parents.

Many people have trouble assuming responsibility for themselves and their life decisions. They shift the responsibility onto fate, their partners, or their parents by conforming to their rules and expectations. They're afraid that they would disappoint or fail if they went their own way. Furthermore, they have *low frustration tolerance*, meaning they can barely endure the negative feelings that result from making a mistake. When we take responsibility for our behavior, after all, on the one side there's the freedom of choice, but on the other is the risk of making the wrong decision and having to live with this "personal failure." In this respect, it's safer for us when our "protectors" tell us what to do.

Since childhood, these people have been accustomed to others calling the shots, to the point that they don't know what they themselves want. They're often unhappy and grouchy, because they end up doing a lot of things they don't actually want to do. They usually act out of a misplaced sense of obligation rather than their own desires or visions. In order to do the latter, they would have to develop a much clearer sense of who they are and what they want.

Some parents apply pressure that borders on blackmail. They might threaten to disown their son or daughter if the kid doesn't follow family rules, leaving the kid with no option but to break from the family if they want to go their own way.

This deters many people who naturally feel a bond with their family. Furthermore, to take such a radical step as this, they would need the central thing their power-hungry parents had quashed in them: a strong sense of self. When parents are overly involved—for better or worse—in their children's life choices, the children come to doubt their ability to make good decisions without Mom and Dad's input.

Similarly, some "power players" will threaten us—their partner—with punishment or separation if we don't do their bidding. We feel too dependent on them to take a real stand or head for the hills. In this scenario, too, our shadow child is terrified it wouldn't make it on its own. What's more, when our self-protection strategy is "I'll remain a child," our shadow child is quick to feel guilt. The shadow child will often feel a certain complicity in difficult situations, something our parents or partner may even encourage. Admitting personal guilt also makes the relationship with our "tormentors" slightly more bearable, as it puts our parents or partner in a better light. By idealizing our relationship with our supposed protectors, we can maintain our dependence on them. This idealization protects us from a tough argument and/or the terror of separation. Assuming a level of supposed complicity can also give us back a feeling of control, or at least reduce our sense of powerlessness. One of my clients, for instance, thought his domineering and manipulative wife was justified in almost every accusation she made against him. She was constantly criticizing and blaming him for her depression and migraines. By agreeing, he was (unknowingly) perpetuating a certain illusion of control. The alternative was to feel at the mercy of these unfair judgments.

Sugarcoating things is closely related to admitting supposed complicity in a problem. When we sugarcoat things, we downplay the extent of our own dependence and come to our partner's or parents' defense. We feel deeply loyal to our loved ones, even if our relationships are difficult. Because of our profound desire for connection and our perceived dependence, we suppress the issues in the relationship with our "protector."

In the past, women were typically expected to be dependent on men in many cultures, which is sometimes still the case. However, there have always been plenty of men who delegate their responsibilities to their partner, expecting that "Mommy" will take care of everything that isn't directly involved in breadwinning—although sometimes that's included, too. More and more men are financially dependent on their partners, not because they're doing more to help raise the children, but because they're unable to gain a foothold in the workplace.

In praise of this strategy: You work very hard to protect your shadow child by trying to do everything right. You put incredible effort into being a "good boy" or a "sweet, well-behaved girl." Because of this, you also do a lot to make your parents proud.

First aid: Your shadow child is inordinately afraid of making mistakes and disappointing others. With the help of your inner adult, let your shadow child know that mistakes are part of life, and that it's allowed to make them. It's important that you strengthen your adult-self. You can accomplish this by practicing the art of argumentation. A good argument is that you are responsible for creating your own joy—as your parents are for creating theirs. You weren't put on this planet to fulfill other people's expectations. Remind yourself that every decision you make takes you one step forward on your life path. If you just stand in one place, it's true that you won't get lost, but you also won't get anywhere. I'll show you how to practice argumentation in the section "Learn to Deal with Conflict and Shape Your Relationships" on page 239.

SELF-PROTECTION STRATEGY:
FLIGHT, WITHDRAWAL, AND AVOIDANCE

Typical beliefs: "I'm at your mercy," "I'm too weak," "I'm worthless," "I'm inferior," "I can't trust you," "Solitude is safe," "I can't do it."

Flight and withdrawal are cherished self-protection strategies when someone wants to avoid a conflict they don't feel up to facing. As I've mentioned several times already, we usually employ multiple self-protection strategies at once, varying them based on circumstance. For instance, we might attack in one situation, but flee in another—it all depends on our estimated chances at success. Furthermore, self-protection strategies such as attack or flight are not problematic, per se, but are instead useful and natural reactions to protect us from threats. The problem lies in the definition of the threat. The weaker and more vulnerable my shadow child feels, the more quickly it will read a situation as dangerous. People who underestimate their capabilities because of their unconscious beliefs often get caught in constant flight. They flee as readily from confrontation with their own fears and supposed weaknesses as they do from confrontation with other people, who bring their own weaknesses into the mix.

People who hole up at home for protection often internalized as a child that being alone was safer than being around others. When we're alone, not only do we feel safe, but we also feel free, because only then do we feel we're allowed to make decisions and act as we please. As soon as other people come close, our childhood programming kicks in, which tells us to fulfill these people's (perceived) expectations. (More on this in the next section.)

Running away from ourselves or others doesn't necessarily mean disappearing into solitude. People can also flee into activities such as work, hobbies, or scrolling through social media. Diving into activities serves the purpose of distracting us from our main problem. We might not even be aware of what we're doing, since these distractions suppress the underlying hardships the shadow child is suffering. Constant activity provides a fantastic distraction from the shadow child's self-doubt and fears. Millions of people can't sit still because in the stillness, their negative beliefs become audible. They stress themselves out and those around them with their restless bustle. The balancing act between healthy and unhealthy is very tricky here, too. "Distraction" can also be a very useful way to get out of a funk. If the distraction causes the actual problem to grow rather than shrink, however, it would be a better idea to face the issue directly. The first step toward accomplishing this is to acknowledge that we have a problem—this is the most important, most fundamental measure in problem solving.

Closely associated with flight and withdrawal is the self-protection strategy of *avoidance*. Every last one of us is happy to avoid unpleasant situations or tasks from time to time. Yet again, it comes down to the question of extent. We often wish to avoid situations and tasks that are scary or unpleasant. The problem with this tactic, however, is that the reluctance and fear we feel become stronger through avoidance, not weaker. The list of unpleasant tasks that I put off grows longer by the day, which only increases my disinclination to tackle it. And the fear becomes more potent the more often I swerve around it. Avoidance simply convinces us more thoroughly that we can't handle the situation. In other words, it's the cerebral confirmation of our feelings of fear and reluctance. Furthermore, avoidance prevents us from discovering that we actually *can* handle a given situation. Conversely, we're especially proud of ourselves when we successfully rise to a challenge—despite our fear. We're then far less fearful the next time around.

A particular form of flight and avoidance is the *impulse to play dead*, in which we flee into ourselves, switching off internally. This process is not typically voluntary, but will instead occur as an automatic, knee-jerk response to a stimulus. This self-protection strategy emerges in the first years of life, when children are unable to either run away or defend themselves. Their one remaining option is to cut off the contact internally in an attempt to feel as little as possible. The technical term for this strategy is *dissociation*.

When feeling overwhelmed by interpersonal contact, people who experience dissociation go offline internally. The person they're speaking with can sense that they're absent inside. People who tend toward dissociation have difficulty setting internal and external boundaries. This means we absorb and feel responsible for the vacillations and attitudes of those around us. Our antennae are permanently set to receive signals, which can cause us great stress in interpersonal situations. Given our perforated internal boundaries, we're quick to feel inundated in the presence of others. We don't rely solely on internal retreat to protect ourselves, but will also withdraw externally. We feel safest when we're alone. The child within us has learned that interpersonal contact means stress. Either because we weren't allowed to distance ourselves from a weak, needy mother or father, or because our parents were a threatening presence. People who have experienced trauma (even as adults) will often demonstrate dissociative tendencies.

In praise of this strategy: It makes sense to flee or withdraw to protect your shadow child when it's feeling overwhelmed. You're taking care of yourself and divvying up your strengths to help.

First aid: Although withdrawal is a very useful self-protection strategy, it can also mean you're often running away from "ghosts." But you really don't need to hide. With the help of the exercises in this book, let your shadow child know that it's adequate and, most important, that it's allowed to assert and defend itself. Once you start advocating for your own rights, desires, and needs, you'll discover that you feel much freer and more self-confident in your interactions with other people.

SIDE NOTE: THE SHADOW CHILD'S FEAR OF CLOSENESS AND BEING MONOPOLIZED

When a child is required to get in line with their parents' expectations, they end up unable to assert themselves properly. Instead, the child learns to put out their receptors to anticipate and respond to their parents' moods and desires. It's especially hard for the child if the parents don't strictly enforce their expectations, but instead express *disappointment* if the child fails to behave according to their wishes. When Mom gets sad because her child fails to meet her expectations, the kid doesn't stand a chance at ever distancing themselves from parental influence. The child feels sorry for their mother and responsible for her sorrow. They then "voluntarily" do whatever Mommy wants, to keep her happy. A child whose mother responds to the same offense with anger, meanwhile, is more likely to think "What a dummy!"—thus establishing some internal distance.

I see many people in my practice who are afraid of commitment. They have a hard time expressing themselves in a healthy manner and are therefore quick to feel crowded by their partner's closeness. In many cases, one of their parents (usually their mother) monopolized them as a child. For instance, she may have been disappointed when the child wanted to play with friends instead of staying home with her. This was the case for thirty-nine-year-old Thomas. When Thomas was a child, his mother had been desperately unhappy in her marriage to his father, who was unloving and unfaithful. She was often sad as a result. Little Thomas tried hard to comfort his poor mom and slipped increasingly into the role of her replacement partner, not least because she would cry to him about his terrible father. Little Thomas sensed that it helped her to have him around. He would often skip out on playing with his friends after school, in order to make his mom happy. He therefore never learned to distance himself from his mother in a healthy manner and leave her to take responsibility for her own problems. Over time, he came to believe that, "I can't leave you," "I'm responsible for your happiness," "I always have to be with you," and "I'm not allowed to have my own free will."

As an adult, because of this mind-set, Thomas could only handle a certain degree of closeness with his partner. As soon as his girlfriend entered the room, he would start to feel like he was losing himself. He only felt truly free and autonomous when he was alone. After moments of closeness, he would therefore reassert a certain distance from his partner. The stress he felt in the presence of any given girlfriend caused his feelings for her to change: initial feelings of love gave way to serious doubts as to whether she was the right one. He often sought refuge in his work, sometimes in flirtation or affairs, or he would end the relationship and look for someone "better." He did this until one day, he realized that his unending search for "the one" had less to do with the supposed shortcomings of his ex-girlfriends than with his own fear of commitment.

Thomas unpacked his mother projections in our psychotherapy sessions and learned that he can still feel like his own person while in a relationship. To accomplish this, he had to learn to assert himself and bring his own desires and needs to the table. The child within him had internalized that relationships were something to be *endured*, but that he couldn't *actively help shape* them. And the more Thomas came to feel that he wasn't at the mercy of his girlfriend but had rights of his own in the relationship, the better able he was to enjoy her closeness, rather than wanting to flee from it.

SPECIAL CASE: DESCENT INTO ADDICTION

Eating, drinking alcohol, smoking, doing drugs, and popping pills all serve to comfort a shadow child in search of protection, security, relaxation, and reward. Shopping, work, play, sex, and sports can also be pursued to the point of addiction, in order to distract ourselves from our concerns and problems. Addiction primarily plays off the sensation of pleasure. Drugs—whether chemical or behavioral—release the neurotransmitter dopamine, also known as the "happiness hormone." When we yield to a craving, we're casting off unpleasantness and producing feelings of pleasure. The substance or behavior immediately rewards us; if we're unable to access our drug, the unpleasant feelings appear in the form of withdrawal symptoms. Our motivation system is based on the experience of pleasure or displeasure, which is what makes it so hard to free ourselves from addiction. After all, we're always looking to avoid pain and feel pleasure in life. We are forever in search of happiness, which makes us susceptible to dependency. The long-term negative consequences won't come until sometime in the future, meaning they can easily be suppressed. Or the addict is already suffering the consequences of their behavior—with fatty liver disease or chronic bronchitis, for instance—but they still can't stop, because the prospect of living without the drug is too scary or physically painful.

Chemical dependencies, such as alcoholism, are considered metabolic diseases by many medical experts today because they alter the brain, with grave impact on the individual's free will. Withdrawal symptoms and cravings can become so extreme that the person's will simply crumbles.

There are other researchers, such as Gene M. Heyman, a psychologist and lecturer at Harvard Medical School, who contend that addiction is not a disease, but instead a "disorder of choice." One plausible argument for this idea is that epidemiological studies have shown that about half of all drug addicts eventually manage to beat their dependency. Individuals suffering from metabolic diseases such as schizophrenia, Alzheimer's disease, or diabetes do not have this option.

Heyman states that addiction is a behavior governed by its outcomes, as opposed to an involuntary behavior triggered by stimuli, such as blinking. Blinking occurs reflexively in response to a stimulus, such as a camera flash. Winking, on the other hand, is voluntary and controlled by mental structures that gauge the outcome of our actions. For instance, a person will assess their likelihood for success if they decide to wink across the bar at someone they find attractive. Along these lines, addiction is subject to the same laws of motivation and decision-making that otherwise regulate our behavior. A further point in favor of this argument is that most addicts will abandon their behavior at the moment the cost of continuing becomes too high. Or the other way around: They won't quit if the cost of abstinence appears greater than the benefits. This is one of the most insidious phenomena of addiction: that the longer the dependency goes on, the less attractive alternative ways of life appear.

With regard to addiction, in particular, a deep schism separates how the inner adult views their dependency and how the shadow child feels about it. It's usually very clear to the inner adult that their behavior is destructive and that they should stop. The shadow child, meanwhile, wants to be rewarded now (!) and feel good immediately (!). Oral fixations—such as eating, drinking, and smoking—have an incredibly comforting and soothing effect on the inner child. Given the deep (albeit unconscious) association with the mother's breast, oral fixations fulfill the needs for nourishment, security, and being provided for, all of which are deeply rooted in childhood. Addictions are not only attractive to the shadow child seeking solace and distraction, but also appeal to the sun child looking for fun, adventure, and excitement. For that reason, it isn't only individuals looking for distraction and relief from their problems who succumb to addiction, but also folks just looking for a good time. The point is, the inner child is naturally inclined to excess. The child always wants to do whatever is most pleasurable. The problem is that pleasure can give way to dependency, because conditioning alters the addict's habits and brain, and they lose control over their behavior. Unfortunately, the longer the addiction persists, the more discouraged the person becomes about recovery. At some point, even their inner adult starts thinking, "I can't do it."

Recovery from addiction is usually successful when long-term benefits outweigh the shadow child's desire for instant gratification. For instance, many drug addicts recover when a positive change occurs in their life, such as a new job or relationship. For this reason, many recovery programs are based on the principle of minimizing the appeal of short-term fulfillment and making long-term goals appear more attractive. A good number of smokers quit after the public smoking ban was passed, because the short-term satisfaction of having a cigarette was significantly diminished by having to go out into the cold and rain to do so. I believe that the most important factor for recovery is to experience feelings that motivate you to change your behavior. For instance, admitting your fears of the long-term consequences of your habit rather than repressing them, as well as anticipating the joy and relief that you'll feel once you quit. In the side note "Self-Reflection Strategies Against Addiction" on page 288, I'll introduce several ways in which you can motivate your inner child and inner adult to abandon their addictions.

In praise of this strategy: Most addictions are a total blast, once you've accustomed yourself to the behavior. Drinking, smoking, eating, etc., are really fun and release tons of pleasurable feelings. Besides, we're surrounded by temptations. It really isn't easy to resist these things all the time. At the end of the day, all you really want is to feel good.

First aid: The problem, unfortunately, is that there's a high price to pay for most addictions, which is why you often feel guilty after indulging. You're caught in a real dilemma: on the one hand, there's the addiction, which will make you happy in the immediate term, while on the other hand, you're afraid of the consequences. The first step is to have some understanding for yourself and your dependency. It's enough that you're suffering from these behaviors—you don't need to load on the self-reproach. Your shadow child is in need, and it needs your loving attention.

SELF-PROTECTION STRATEGY: NARCISSISM

Typical beliefs: "I'm worthless," "I'm a nobody," "I'm a shitty person," "I'm a loser," "I'm not allowed to have feelings," "I need to do things on my own," "I can never get enough."

According to Greek mythology, the strapping young lad Narcissus fell in love with himself when he spotted his reflection in a pool of water. He suffered from this insatiable self-love until he died. A narcissist is thus a self-obsessed individual who thinks they're the most amazing and important person in the room. This outward demonstration of grandeur and flawlessness, however, is nothing more than a self-protection strategy that a person develops in order not to feel the presence of their injured shadow child.

People with a narcissistic personality learned early in life to suppress their shadow child, which felt worthless and miserable, by adopting an ideal second self. Narcissists do whatever it takes to elevate themselves above the average, to create this *ideal self.* They go to unbelievable lengths to be something special, because their shadow child feels the exact opposite. In order to contain their shadow child, they strive for outsize accomplishments, for power, beauty, success, and recognition. Narcissism thus encompasses a host of self-protection strategies, including, unfortunately, the denigration of other people. Narcissists have an eagle eye for weakness in others, which they're quick to call out. They cannot stand weakness in themselves, nor can they tolerate it in others. By focusing on others, however, their own shortcomings disappear from view. Their criticism elicits the same feelings in the people around them that they hope to avoid themselves: deep insecurity and inferiority. Victim-offender reversal is particularly pronounced with narcissists.

Some narcissists employ the opposite strategy to build themselves up: they idealize those around them. In this case, they show off with their amazing partner, their terrific kids, and their important friends. Many narcissists will also do both, idealizing and denigrating. Oftentimes, a new acquaintance or love interest will first be idealized, then denigrated, and ultimately dumped.

Regardless of which category the narcissist falls into—idealizing or denigrating—they all like to boast about their skills, possessions, and undertakings. This isn't necessarily done with great fanfare and noise. There are also *quiet narcissists*—quite often intellectuals—who discreetly put their superiority and uniqueness on display.

Narcissists do have some endearing qualities, too. They can be incredibly charming, lovable, and interesting. Some are downright charismatic. Their ambition frequently translates into great professional success and respect. Their efforts to be something special often pay off, casting a sort of spell over other narcissists as well as those who exhibit dependent behavioral habits. Relationships between two active narcissists are a roller-coaster ride of passion and mutual injury.

When the narcissist's partner is more dependent in nature, they'll often endure verbal attacks without much resistance and are anxious to please. An undertaking doomed to failure, because regardless of how "good" they've been, their behavior won't alter the narcissist's distorted perception. This distortion combines the narcissist's sweeping suppression of their own weaknesses with an ultra-magnified view of their partner's minor (or imagined) flaws. When a narcissist gets caught up in this way of thinking, their focus narrows and all they see, for instance, is their partner's nose—just a little too big—while all his or her merits fade into the background. This supposed weakness infuriates the narcissist, because their partner is meant to enhance their own position or image. Their partner needs to be perfect, just like them.

No one stands a chance against a narcissist's eye for weakness. Dependent partners can't help but think, though, that if they could just find a way to be better or prettier, the narcissist would be pleased with them. The shadow child frequently arrives at this false conclusion, and not only in relationships with narcissistic personalities. Many people are upset by criticism, however unfair and off the mark it may be. Because of their inner influences, these people are hounded by feelings of guilt and inadequacy. This is even the case when the person's inner adult is well aware of the fact that they're dating a narcissist, and that it isn't their fault when their partner insults them. Their shadow child, however, doesn't realize this, and remains consumed by feelings of inferiority that are perpetually reinforced by the narcissist's comments. The shadow child is desperate for the narcissist's approval in order to heal, and will try even harder to please them. The narcissist doesn't change, though. The dependent partner will see themselves as ineffective and powerless, which further hardens their feelings of dependency. A vicious cycle.

Narcissists make for unpopular colleagues and bosses, given their extreme ambition and power-hungriness. Their irritability further hampers interactions with them: on the outside, it's surprising to see how offended narcissists get over seemingly innocuous things, especially since they seem so unflappable. Their deeply insecure and insulted shadow child doesn't withdraw in sorrow when it feels hurt, though—it becomes insanely angry. Fury and rancor are the narcissist's defining emotions. They can also fall into a deep depression whenever their recipes for success fail and they experience a personal setback. Their shadow child spirals into desperation, because it senses the full extent of its inadequacy and badness. To protect the shadow child, the adult will employ the old strategies to become successful again. The psychological strain can become so severe, however, that some people may start seeing a therapist to get help, or may end up taking their own life. If all goes well in therapy, the narcissist will learn to accept and comfort their shadow child, so that it feels understood and valued, even without having to accomplish something special.

Narcissism is a self-protection strategy that we all use—the degree to which the strategy is employed determines when someone can be called a "narcissist." We all exhibit these behaviors to a lesser degree: We want to look as good as possible, and may sometimes denigrate others to help us achieve this. We may like to boast a little occasionally, and no one can turn their back entirely on the allure of prestige. Our focus may zoom in on other people's shortcomings from time to time, and we may feel embarrassed when our partner "disgraces" us.

We try as hard as we can to hide our weaknesses, and not to feel our shadow child.

In praise of this strategy: You exert tremendous effort to perform well and look good. This requires an incredible amount of power and initiative. You've probably enjoyed a great deal of success in life, and you can be proud of that.

First aid: Your self-protection strategy requires a lot of energy and constantly leads to stressful situations with the people around you. Be aware of the fact that all your efforts to be something special won't heal your shadow child. You can only heal your shadow child once you fully accept it. Stop fighting your supposed weaknesses and accept that you are simply human, like everyone else. Only then will you be able to relax—for maybe the first time in your life.

SELF-PROTECTION STRATEGY: DISGUISE, ROLE-PLAY, AND LIES

Typical beliefs: "I'm not allowed to be this way," "I need to adjust," "I'm bad," "I'm inadequate," "No one loves me," "I'm worthless."

Everybody more or less subscribes to social norms and rules, and exerts some effort to adjust as required. In daily life, we perform countless social rituals without a second thought. We can't be fully open and authentic at all times and with everyone we meet, nor would we want to be. A certain level of restraint and "disguise" to protect ourselves is healthy, natural, and socially acceptable. Some people, however, play defined roles and hide behind a mask. In interactions with others, people who aren't in touch with their feelings or their shadow child often perceive themselves as a "shell." A client once told me that when he went to work in the morning, he regarded himself as "Man in suit goes to office." This client could barely feel his own presence and once described himself as a "human performer." It was as though his shadow child were expressly designed to adjust and satisfy the expectations of other people. Individuals with this problem often say that in interpersonal situations, they "simply function." They reel off a practiced set of behaviors, play a role, and hide behind a mask. They don't dare be authentic. Their fear of rejection and falling prey to attack is extreme. Meanwhile, they don't usually show any outward signs of insecurity.

Even people who are in decent touch with themselves and their feelings often think they need to play a particular role in the company of others. They conceal their own needs and orient themselves to the needs of those around them. Some people can't even leave the house when they're having a bad day, because they feel so vulnerable. They only want to show the world their strong, happy side. This self-protection strategy overlaps considerably with perfectionism and keeping the peace.

People who can't leave the house without their mask feel

the burden of keeping up appearances. Their fear of rejection, were they to reveal more of themselves, is stronger than the suffocation inside the mask. Their shadow child is programmed to adjust and conform. Many people don't even dare to be authentic with their partner. They think they need to keep some parts hidden. As much as possible, they prefer to show their partner their "presentable self" only. They believe that, if they were to be authentic and up-front about their desires and needs, it would place too much strain on the relationship. The very opposite is the case, though: authenticity is what makes a relationship exciting and lively.

This role-playing has the potential to bring relationships to a standstill, exacerbated by the partners' shared aversion to conflict. Both feel such pressure to conform that neither ventures to formulate their own personal needs. Over time, they come to feel as though they're chronically coming up short in the relationship, which causes frustration, but—wanting to avoid conflict—they keep it bottled up inside, where it eats away at them. This cold rage keeps building, which causes the person's feelings for their partner to cool down, too. The relationship becomes rigid and bleak. Eventually the spark peters out entirely, and the relationship ends, with scarcely a harsh word exchanged.

People who habitually adjust themselves to others and adopt different roles cannot be considered sincere. To do so, they would have to lower their defenses and stand by their desires and opinions. Even if they aren't necessarily actively lying, it can be hard for other people to tell where they stand. It also isn't fair if they end a friendship or romantic relationship without providing the other person with a reason. It's equally unfair, however, to present the other person with a "final reckoning" at the end of the relationship, when barely any complaints had been made before. I've often been surprised by the fervor with which people will describe themselves as sincere and honest, but who at the same time shy away from speaking openly with their partner or a good friend.

In praise of this strategy: You do your best to be loved and acknowledged. You put incredible effort into showing only your best side. You're highly skilled at adjusting to different scenarios and have great self-control.

First aid: Your shadow child is quite despondent. It thinks that it somehow needs to be different in order to be loved. Tell your shadow child that that's nonsense. Your inner adult should treat it lovingly and gently, so that it feels safer simply being itself. In smaller settings, practice standing by who you are, what you believe, and what you desire. You'll be amazed at how well other people receive you.

And there we have it: an overview of the most important self-protection strategies. As I wrote at the beginning, it's important that you recognize your individual self-protection strategies that may not have appeared in this list. You've probably also realized that our self-protection strategies are usually the actual cause of our problems. The following exercise is designed to help.

• • •

Exercise: Find Your Personal Self-Protection Strategies

It's possible that your self-protection strategies vary between the different parts of your life. For instance, you may protect yourself from attack at work by perfectly meeting every demand, whereas you can be petty and often pick fights at home. Usually, though, we have a set of standard self-protection strategies that we use in every difficult situation or for any problem we encounter. For instance, perfectionists typically strive to be perfect in every aspect of their lives. Other people, meanwhile, respond to most problems with withdrawal and avoidance. This is why we'll often perceive both our own self-protection strategies and those of others as a kind of personality trait. When someone protects themselves by means of retreat and role-play, for instance, we describe them as withdrawn. Narcissism is also closely associated with the personality of the person in question.

Most people also exhibit certain beliefs that are themselves self-protection strategies, such as "I always have to be nice and well-behaved" or "I'm not allowed to make mistakes."

In order to quickly identify your primary self-protection strategies, simply think back to two or three situations from the past few weeks in which you weren't feeling your best and may have thought, "This is a problem!" Maybe it was a conflict at work, or a situation with your partner in which they annoyed, angered, or otherwise threw you off course. This little memory exercise will help you recognize which situations are more or less typical and likely to cause you frequent difficulties. By referencing these situations, you should be able to observe your self-protection strategies at play. Do you snap into attack mode? Do you withdraw? Do you conform?

Please write down your personal self-protection strategies around the feet of your child drawing (see shadow child image inside the front cover). Formulate them in complete sentences and be as concrete as possible. For instance, do not simply write "Withdrawal," but instead write, "I avoid conflicts," or "I dither and conceal my opinions," or "I seek refuge online." Self-protection strategies can be described by means of concrete behaviors. They're part of what we do. For this reason, I want you to formulate your individual self-protection strategies very specifically, such as, "I go into the garage and mess around on my car," or "I go shopping," or "I fabricate stories—I lie."

Once you've added your self-protection strategies to your child drawing, you'll have right in front of you that part of your psyche that's always causing you problems: your shadow child.

THE SHADOW CHILD IS ALWAYS THERE

As we've discussed, all the problems we face in life that hinge on some level of personal involvement can be traced back to the shadow child. There's nothing more to it. It's just a matter of theme and variation. Most people have a hard time believing this, though. And it really isn't easy to grasp that in most cases, hiding behind our problems—seemingly *so* diverse and *so* complicated—is the shadow child with its simple beliefs. I experience this time and again with my patients.

For example, Billie, twenty-seven, comes to her tenth therapy session and tells me about a problem she had in the past week with her best friend. When I respond that this information is already in her child illustration, she acts surprised. We review her beliefs and self-protection strategies, and she's amazed to realize (yet again!) that we're always looking at variations of the same theme. In Billie's case, because of her shadow child's feelings of inferiority that stem from the belief "I'm inadequate," she gets offended by the slightest criticism and responds by withdrawing.

Even if I've already become acquainted with my shadow child, I can still easily overlook it in my everyday life and not catch myself when I start viewing the world through its eyes again, operating according to my old patterns. In other words, you can lose sight of yourself and end up falling for your own projections.

YOUR REALITY IS WHAT YOU MAKE IT

If you're looking to break from your childhood programming—read: to become happier—you must acknowledge the fact that you, together with your shadow child and its beliefs, construct your own reality. This means that your problems—provided they're not uncontrollable twists of fate—result from your subjective perception of yourself and your surroundings. *The one thing you have to understand is that you are free to reshape your own perception, thoughts, and feelings.* You probably don't believe me. After all, we so often experience our feelings as forceful and inescapable. And starting in childhood, we're accustomed to there being only *one*—that is, *our*—reality. For this reason, I want you to deliberately examine how extensively your negative beliefs influence your feelings, and how extensively your self-protection strategies permeate your everyday life.

The reason these childhood systems have such a deep impact and operate like a subjective lens can be attributed to the fact that our brains learn through *conditioning:* the more often we have a thought, perform an action, or experience a feeling, the more real these things become, as the neuronal stimulus-response link created in our brain, or our consciousness, deepens. The more often the neuronal connections in our brains are fed by the habitual repetition of thoughts, feelings, and behaviors, the wider they become, expanding into data superhighways, whereas the space for alternative thoughts, feelings, and behaviors is limited to a tiny footpath, at best.

Once more for good measure: You construct your reality yourself, and this process will continue to run automatically and unconsciously—until you notice it. As soon as you do, you'll be able to alter your reality, along with your thoughts, feelings, and behaviors. This is current brain science, not some esoteric exercise. The next chapters are dedicated to bringing about this change and taking a constructive and appropriate approach to designing your own reality. Before we turn to the sun child and its self-reflection strategies, we'll want to take some time to embrace and console—and maybe even help—our poor, injured shadow child.

In addition to the exercises in the following sections, you can download the imaginary journey *The Shadow Child Meditation* from stefaniestahl.com.

Heal Your Shadow Child

The biggest concern we face in life, the one that causes us the most anguish, is that we'll make a mistake or wrong decision. We strive to be right about things and behave correctly. We struggle to forgive our own mistakes. For many people, it's not just about the mistakes they make—they see *themselves* as a mistake. They have the subliminal feeling that they're inadequate and need to be different, somehow. This feeling is the result of the shadow child and its negative beliefs. That poor child. It leads a miserable existence, thinking there's something wrong with it. The child feels misunderstood and abandoned by the grown-ups—that is, by the inner adult. Just like it used to feel with Mom and Dad (and maybe even other kids) who didn't understand it. But the less accepted the shadow child feels, the worse off it is. It's high time your shadow child felt your consolation and understanding.

In the following sections, I'd like to introduce a few practical exercises for you to heal, or at least console, your shadow child. As I've said, it's extremely important that you and your inner adult understand that all those nasty little statements and feelings are simply the product of childhood influences and do not represent reality. You may not entirely believe me yet, but I'm doing everything I can to help you realize this over the course of this book.

We now know that we'll often injure ourselves and sometimes other people because of our shadow child and its self-protection strategies. It is thus very important that we separate the shadow child from our adult-self, which allows us to better regulate and control ourselves. This requires us to *catch ourselves* whenever we start feeling things and behaving from the stance of our shadow child. It's only when we catch ourselves that we're able to snap out of "shadow child mode" and switch over to our adult-self. The following exercises therefore focus on regulating our perception, thinking, and feelings. In other words, they're about *self-management*.

It's important that you accept responsibility for your own process of change, which means that you participate in the following exercises and practice them in your daily life. The more often you do, the more your brain will absorb this new programming and these positive feelings. It's like learning a dance: You have to concentrate really hard at first, and everything feels awkward. Over time, however, the movements become locked into your body memory, until they flow automatically.

* * *

Exercise: Find Inner Helpers

In one of my workshops, a participant shared that it was really hard to take on all these challenges by himself. He simply wished he had someone by his side in tough situations. My dear friend and fellow coach Karin assured him that he didn't need to face these situations alone. She then told the story of her friend Rahmée, who was born in Cameroon and moved to Germany with her family as a young child. Today she's a successful businesswoman. When heading into negotiations with her German and international colleagues, she never goes in alone: standing behind her are her grandmother, the family matriarch; her grandfather, the tribal elder; and her uncle, the shaman of her village. This image gives her the strength she needs to steel herself for the judgments some negotiating partners may unfortunately still have because of her skin color.

This self-reinforcement is as obvious as it is magical, which is why I'd like to pass it on to you: find your own inner helpers and supporters, who will stand by you in times of need. It might be a single person, or a whole team, like Rahmée had. You can conjure up real people, even if they've already passed away. But you can also call upon imaginary characters for help, such as a fairy godmother or Superman. Allow your helpers to emerge from your imagination. You may even use different helpers, depending on the situation, their skills, and your need.

Whenever you need support, imagine that these individuals are accompanying you on your way. Try it out in the following exercises.

* * *

Exercise: Strengthen Your Adult-Self

In order to heal your shadow child, you need a strong, sturdy inner adult. A resilient inner adult understands that your negative beliefs are simply the result of childhood influences. Our rational mind has the ability to make logical arguments. Arguments are like a load-bearing structure with which we strengthen ourselves and find security. I'll return to this image repeatedly. First, a few arguments, or rather facts, that you can consider in order to create a little distance between your shadow child and your adult-self.

- No child is born bad. Children cannot be bad people.
- Children can be annoying and exhausting, but this has no bearing on their value. It is the parents' responsibility—

before they become parents—to consider whether they want to take on the stress of parenthood.

- Children *have to be* annoying, in fact. They're more or less powerless, after all, and they need some way to prompt adults to satisfy their fundamental needs. Children's MO: Survive! Grow up! Learn!

- If parents are overwhelmed by the task of raising their children, they should seek assistance. The kids can't help being kids.

- Children have the right to have their emotional and physical needs met. Their parents are responsible for this.

- Feelings and needs are fundamentally normal and correct, although children must learn not to express these things every time they feel the urge.

- It is the parents' duty to understand their children's feelings and needs. It is not the children's responsibility to understand and satisfy the feelings and needs of their parents.

- It is the parents' duty to love their children and make them feel welcome in this world. Children should not feel they have to behave in a certain way to make their parents love them.

- Much of what can be exhausting in children (wide-ranging interests, perseverance, etc.) is admired in adults. As such, it is the parents' duty to bear with these behaviors or traits for a time, and to steer them in the right direction. Trying to quash these tendencies is a sign of incompetence.

You are free to have thoughts like these, based entirely on your personal history, beliefs, and current situation. Practice the art of argumentation. As we've discussed, arguments provide the inner adult with support and strength.

Good tip: When thinking or speaking about yourself, try to get in the habit of creating a little distance between your problem and yourself. Instead of thinking, "*I* am afraid of being rejected, abandoned, ridiculed, etc." say to yourself, "*The shadow child within me* is afraid . . ." I practice this often with my clients, and it truly does help to put a little wedge between yourself and your problem. This phrasing prevents you from identifying wholly and completely with your shadow child.

● ● ●

Exercise: Accept the Shadow Child

It is a psychological law that we experience more stress and strain the more we fight against ourselves. Many people spend their existence in permanent battle with themselves. It's both exhausting and futile. Self-acceptance is the prerequisite for relaxation and productive growth. To avoid any misunderstandings: Self-acceptance doesn't mean I have to like everything about myself. Self-acceptance means saying yes to what's there. It's the opposite of self-loathing and self-deception. Self-acceptance means accepting that my feelings—the good and the bad—are part of me. It also means acknowledging my strengths along with my limitations. It is only once I have acknowledged these things that I can accept and—if I so choose—work on them. After all, self-acceptance doesn't imply stasis.

For the following exercise, please close your eyes and establish an internal connection to your shadow child. You can do this by internally reciting your negative beliefs and tapping into the feelings they provoke. Or it may be easier for you to call up your shadow child by thinking of a situation in which it was (or is) very active. Perhaps a situation from childhood in which you felt ashamed, misunderstood, lonely, or unfairly treated. Or maybe a time in your adult life in which your shadow child felt just terrible. Feel what you're feeling. You're probably encountering long-known companions, such as fear, insecurity, sorrow, pressure, or rage. Establish a connection to these feelings, breathe deeply in and out of your belly, and say to yourself: "Yes, there it is, that's my shadow child. Here's how it is, my dear shadow child. You're allowed to be here, just as you are. I welcome you."

You'll discover that the more you accept your shadow child, the quieter it will become. It finally feels seen, accepted, and understood.

* * *

Exercise: Consoling the Shadow Child

We're going to go a little further in the next exercise. This time, your adult-self is going to help the shadow child understand that its negative beliefs and feelings are the result of flawed programming.

For this exercise, your inner adult is going to adopt a very sympathetic, parental attitude toward the shadow child. It might help to look at an old childhood photo of yourself. If you have a hard time mustering this loving attitude toward your shadow child, imagine that you are speaking with a scared little kid. He might be afraid the other kids don't want to play with him. How would you comfort him? By saying, "Don't be so stupid!," or by encouraging him, holding his hand, and walking with him over to the group? Probably the latter. You can tap into this generous, friendly attitude when dealing with your shadow child as well. In other words, practice goodwill toward yourself. Goodwill is not only the essence of every interpersonal connection, but is also critical to making peace between your shadow child and yourself.

From this benevolent inner place, you will now address the shadow child in a friendly tone. It's fine to speak loudly—this is often more effective. If this makes you feel a bit silly, you can also deliver your speech in your mind.

1. The inner adult explains to the shadow child how things were back then with Mommy and Daddy, which might go a little something like this (of course, using details from your own life): "Oh, sweetheart, you poor thing. You didn't have it easy back then with Mommy and Daddy. Mommy was always so tired and stressed. And she was sick all the time. You always got the feeling that things were too much for Mommy to handle. You always tried to be good, so that you wouldn't be a burden on her, too. But you could never make Mommy really happy. She was usually sad. And Daddy was no help. He was always bickering with Mommy, and with you, too, a lot of the time. But when he was in a good mood, he could be really fun. Those moments made you so happy, and all you wanted was for his good mood to stick. But it never did, and it was only a matter of time before he started arguing with Mommy again. And because Mommy and Daddy were so unhappy together, and were always so stressed and overwhelmed as a result, you reached some pretty silly conclusions. You thought, 'I'm not enough,' 'I always have to be good,' or 'I'm a burden' . . . " (At this point, please read the core beliefs you determined for yourself earlier.)

2. When speaking with your shadow child, please use a child's vocabulary, so that the child within you feels you

are addressing it directly. If your mother was very dominant, for instance, remember that the term "dominant" is
drawn from adult vocabulary. Translate it into language
a child would understand, such as saying that Mommy
was "bossy." Words like "depressed" or "aggressive" aren't
within a child's vocabulary, either, and should be re-
placed with terms like "sad" or "mad."

3. Next, you will deliver the important message to your
shadow child that none of this was its fault, and it would
have developed much different convictions if Mommy and
Daddy hadn't been so overwhelmed. You could say something along the lines of: "It's very important to me that
you understand that none of this was your fault. Mommy
and Daddy made mistakes—not you! And if Mommy and
Daddy hadn't been so worn out, or if you'd had different
parents, you would realize that you're enough just the way
you are. You would know that your parents are very proud
of you. They love you, even if you're naughty sometimes
and just do what you want to do. And it's okay if you're a
burden sometimes, too—they're happy to take care of
you when you need them to."

You can adapt these statements to match your own
problems and negative beliefs. It's not about using this
text verbatim. Rather, it's about understanding the principle that with the help of your adult-self, you can explain

to your shadow child that its beliefs are rather arbitrary and have nothing—*nothing*—to do with your real worth.

You can, of course, also do this exercise if you had a mostly happy childhood and your parents only made a few mistakes. Open the conversation by explaining to your shadow child, "My darling shadow child, Mommy and Daddy did a lot right, and we're very happy with them, but they could have done a little more/a little less here..."

From now on, it's very important that your shadow child no longer be allowed to take control of your actions. Your shadow child may be fearful or despondent, or want to run away or lash out. But the adult calls the shots. It's like in real life with small children. If a child is afraid of going to the dentist, her loving parent will hold her hand and help her cope with the visit. The adult won't let the child call the shots and cancel the appointment. Just like they won't let her skip school when she doesn't feel like going. You can approach your shadow child in the same way: listen to it and allow it to describe its fears and concerns. Ultimately, though, you're the one making the rational decisions about what's going to happen.

You should speak often with your shadow child—as often as it takes for the message to get through. It doesn't always need to be a long discussion. If you come face-to-face with a difficult situation in your everyday life, for instance, and catch yourself reeling off negative beliefs or slipping into fear, rage, or desperation, it can help to just reach out to your shadow child and pat it on the head to encourage or comfort it. You can also say a few words to console or cheer it up. This gesture creates some distance between your childhood mind-set and adult reality, and prevents the former from running on autopilot. The slight distance created between your shadow child's perception and your inner adult allows you to reflect upon your own patterns. This provides the opportunity to reach new decisions regarding your behavior.

● ● ●

Exercise: Catch Yourself and Switch

"Catch yourself and switch"—I like to refer to this as the "Steffi Stahl mantra." Catch yourself and switch is the queen of self-help strategies. What it comes down to is catching myself whenever the shadow child takes hold and immediately releasing myself from its grasp by switching back to my adult-self. This action catapults me back into my current reality. I know plenty of people who have changed their lives using this exercise alone, yet it's as simple as it is fundamental.

The idea behind this little exercise came to me while watching a 4-D film at Bavaria Film Studio in Munich a few years back. We were all wearing the standard 3-D glasses as we watched an animated clip of sledding in winter. But in addition to the 3-D visual, the seats shook and wind blew in our faces to create the 4-D effect. It was the perfect illusion—everyone in the audience felt like they were seated at the front of the sled. I'm sure you can imagine how "hellish" a ride it was! The entire theater was screaming. It only lasted about five minutes, and when it was over, I thought: "That's exactly it!" Had I wanted to break the spell of fear during the screening, I would have had to enlist my adult-self to shift from the field perspective ("I'm on a sled") to the observer perspective ("I'm in a movie theater"). From the observer perspective, I would have perceived that the fear was generated by nothing more than a projection on the screen and some practical effects; I was safe and sound in my seat.

When you find yourself governed by your shadow child, it means you're looking at things from the field perspective. You believe everything you think and feel. In other words, it's your very own 4-D sledding experience. From the observer perspective, meanwhile, you would realize you're actually safe and sound, and the fear is a projection from the past. You might therefore come to recognize that the people in your life often function as moving screens onto which you project your fears. Here's an example: Ron, forty-five, is an engineer. He's sitting in a team meeting and has a fantastic suggestion he'd like to make. He doesn't dare to, though, because the solution he has in mind is pretty unconventional, and he's afraid his teammates will reject it. But then he catches himself. He realizes that this trepidation comes straight from his shadow child (one of his core beliefs is "Nobody takes me seriously," which manifests in a fear of rejection—a standard shadow child feeling). The moment he catches himself, he releases himself from this feeling by switching back to his adult-self, briefly comforting his shadow child (by giving its hand a warm squeeze), and returning to his current reality, in which he is a brilliant engineer and his colleagues are *not* his mom and dad. Grown-up Ron raises his hand, ready to share his idea immediately.

Most important is that we practice *attentiveness to ourselves*. Two things are required here: First, the explicit decision to accept *responsibility* for ourselves and our feelings, thus allowing us to quit playing the victim. Second, the *mental discipline* to avoid getting bogged down by the shadow child. Instead, by being attentive to ourselves, we float overhead and *notice* whenever we retreat to our shadow child.

To accomplish this, establish and adopt a *meta-stance*. What does that mean? It means that, once and for all, you are going to accept the fact that your shadow child is a pure projection from childhood. Then keep a close eye on yourself, and whenever necessary, remember: catch yourself and switch. You'll find that over time, your shadow child will have less and less to say.

* * *

Exercise: Overwrite Old Memories

As we have discovered, the experiences we had with our parents or other caretakers leave their mark upon our memories. These memories are encoded in our mind, in the connections between our synapses. Sometimes all it takes is a tiny trigger to be sent spinning into old memories, even if you're not consciously aware this is happening—just think of Michael and Sarah and the forgotten chips. Some memories are burned so deeply into our mind that we will quickly and repeatedly fall back on old patterns. We can recast these images, however. *Our mind does not differentiate very clearly between imagination and reality.* For instance, if we want to feel fear, all we need to do is imagine a stressful situation, such as an upcoming exam. In the same way, you can use your power of imagination to recast negative memories—the mind is able to overwrite them, a practice that helps in self-healing past wounds. This overwriting allows us to change the past to a certain extent, and with it, the negative feelings it can arouse. As the German author and poet Erich Kästner once said, "It's never too late to have a good childhood."

The next exercise is used in schema therapy, and I have borrowed it from the book *Schema Therapy in Practice*, by Arnoud Arntz and Gitta Jacob.

You probably remember at least one, if not several, situations in childhood that were "unfav'rable." They may even have been oppressive, frightening, or—worst case—traumatizing. Situations that may have been typical of your parents' or caretakers' approach to childrearing.

1. Please select a concrete situation from your youth that is closely tied to the characteristics of your shadow child. If this memory triggers debilitating feelings, it is not necessary to immerse yourself fully in it. For instance, if one of your parents abused you, it's enough to simply imagine them raising their hand—you do not need to replay the entire scene. You should, however, adopt the "field perspective," meaning you're not experiencing the memory from the outside, but are instead viewing it through the eyes of the child you were at the time.

2. Feel exactly what you felt at the time—but again, you don't need to fully immerse yourself in the sensation. If you were terrified, for instance, it's more than enough to just experience a little fear.

3. Using your imagination, picture the moment of your rescue. In other words, conjure up a helper who appears on the scene. This helper can be anyone you choose. It can be a real person, such as a beloved aunt or grandmother, or it can be a fictional character, such as Superman or a fairy godmother. Your imagination is allowed

free rein in these exercises. Even you, in adult form, can show up to intervene in the situation. Here are a few suggestions for ways in which you can overwrite the situation for yourself:

- If your caretaker was often stressed out or agitated, imagine that your helper appears and explains to them that they aren't allowed to take it out on you. Your caretaker is sent to see a psychotherapist, and from now on, you're always joined by a kind fairy who protects you.
- If your caretaker was threatening, imagine that the police or an action hero shows up and throws them in jail.
- If your caretaker was often sad and depressed, with the result that you had to look after them as a child, imagine that someone from child protective services stops by. This person assures you—child that you are—that you can go play, and they'll look after your parent. You, the child, thus gain a reliable and protective figure in your life; again, this individual may be drawn from the real world or from your imagination.
- If your caretaker was super strict and demanding, your helper can explain that children need to be praised sometimes, too, and can show your caretaker how to better empathize with you. In this case, your caretaker gains a coach who sticks with them and helps protect you, the child.

You can use the powers of your imagination in this way to create a happy ending for yourself. This exercise also works very well on painful memories that have nothing to do with your parents.

* * *

Exercise: Connection and Security for the Shadow Child

This exercise is aimed at the need for love and connection that both children and adults experience. In your mind, you're going to amplify the positive bonding moments you had with your parents or other close relatives. Dive into the memory of those really nice, close, loving, cuddly, and tender moments you experienced with your caretakers. Immerse yourself in this happy place and open up lots of space for feelings of security, certainty, and simply being in good hands. Really feel that sense of connection, the sense that you were deeply loved and welcome in this moment.

If you don't have any memory of close moments with your parents or other relatives, you can pick out imaginary parents. In your imagination, give yourself the parents you could have used as a child—they can be real people, such as the parents of a close friend, or imaginary figures. Close your eyes, and let your unconscious give you loving parents.

Picture how happy your new parents are with you. Allow

them to behave exactly as you would have wanted as a child. Give yourself a new home. You can summon your new parents any time you need them.

* * *

Exercise: Write Your Shadow Child a Letter

It can help to look at a childhood picture of yourself for this exercise. You're going to write your shadow child a letter, just as a loving mom or dad would write to their child to make them feel better when they're down. For example:

My darling Rosie,

You are such a good little girl, and I'm very proud of you. And I'm so sorry that you always worry so much about your body. You don't need to be perfect for me! I love you exactly the way you are. I think you're beautiful in so many ways. In my eyes, you're the sweetest girl I know. Please stop comparing yourself to the models you see on TV and in magazines. Take a look around, out on the street or at the pool, till you realize that very few women and girls look like the ones you see in fashion magazines. Stop driving yourself crazy!

Love you lots,

Big, grown-up Rosie

Here's another one:

Hey Johnny,

You worry about everything. You're terrified of failure and losing your social footing, so you're constantly going full-throttle both at work *and* in your free time. I want to tell you something: you don't always need to overextend yourself like this. You're enough exactly the way you are. And you do things so well that you can afford to loosen up a little. All your stupid beliefs, like "I'm inadequate" and "I've got to manage this alone," those are all from back then, from Mom and Dad. I mean, you really didn't have it easy growing up. Mom was always stressed out, and Dad was barely ever home. You tried so hard to make Mom happy, but it never really worked. She was always exhausted and miserable. You thought this meant you had to be an even better little boy, so you threw yourself into your schoolwork. But listen, it wasn't your fault that Mom was always in such a foul mood! She should have gotten help back then. She probably should have seen a therapist. You know she was overwhelmed because her own shadow child was so insecure. Mom always thought she was inadequate. But you couldn't help that! And the world looks different now—we're grown up and free. Let's finally just enjoy life! You don't always have to be the best. Relax, and go play soccer again sometime—

you always loved that. Start having more fun. It's much better for you than your daily grind.

Love,

Johnny

* * *

Exercise: Understanding Your Shadow Child

The following exercise should also help you differentiate your shadow child's perception from that of your inner adult, thus granting you more freedom in your decisions and actions.

1. For this exercise, take a concrete problem you're having with yourself or another person. Then place two chairs facing each other. Sit down on one and deliberately channel your shadow child. Fully inhabiting your shadow child's perspective, start describing your problem. Allow the shadow child to speak about its feelings and beliefs related to the issue. Pay close attention to what your problem sounds like and how it feels to describe and experience it from this perspective.

2. Now cut off your shadow child and deliberately summon your inner adult. If you need to "shake off" your shadow child, try jumping around or patting down your body. Fully inhabiting your inner adult mind-set, switch seats. From this position, observe the shadow child that was

just sitting across from you, and analyze your problem with your own critical, rational mind.

Here's an example: Babs suffers from panic attacks. She's afraid to walk or drive from point A to point B because she's afraid she'll lose control and faint. I ask Babs to channel her shadow child completely and describe her problem from that place.

Her shadow child: "When I imagine going out by myself, I immediately panic. I feel small and helpless. I'm terrified I'll fall down. That would be so embarrassing. I might even die. No one will help me. I want my mommy to come and stay by my side. I can't do it alone!"

I now ask Babs to switch seats and channel her adult-self instead.

Her adult-self: "I see a little girl who's afraid to stand on her own two feet. Objectively speaking, though, nothing could even happen if she did faint, which is totally unlikely, I'm sure that passersby would come to her aid. No, I think the actual problem is that the little one thinks she can't find her way without Mommy. I can see now that she hasn't detached at all from her parents. She wants someone to look after her and take over her responsibilities. She doesn't feel independent or capable of facing the challenges of life. I think I need to take better care of her, listen more often to how she's actually feeling..."

The chair dialogue reveals to Babs that her phobia of leaving the house alone is rooted in a host of old childhood fears. She realizes that she's been suppressing her shadow child, who has been yearning for affection and support. This discovery allows her to reflect upon her own inadequate liberation from her parents and to work on becoming more independent and self-confident.

It's hard for most people to truly separate their inner child from their inner adult. For instance, they'll use adult vocabulary while speaking from the child's perspective, using expressions that a little kid would never say—and the other way around. That was the case with Babs at first (I summarized and cleaned up the chair dialogue above). For instance, while channeling her shadow child, Babs said, "I know that my fears are exaggerated." This rational assessment came straight from her adult-self. And while adopting her adult perspective, she said, "I just wanna go hide away at home"—a wish that clearly originated with her shadow child. You might chime in here, "Well, why can't grown-up Babs also want to go hide away at home?" It's because this desire is the result of her shadow child's fear of being unable to cope with the world out there. Grown-up Babs actually really likes being around people, but she's saddled with these fears.

It isn't always easy to distinguish between the child and adult parts of ourselves. For that reason, it's important that you truly speak and feel like a kid when channeling your shadow child. And when you take up the adult position, be mindful of analyzing your problem in a sober, unemotional way.

This exercise can also be done in writing, which sometimes makes it easier to keep the two parts separate.

* * *

Exercise: The Three Positions of Perception

This exercise ties in closely to the preceding one, but view it less as an "exercise" and more as a tool for structuring your reality. The three positions of perception provide solid ground from which you can solve your problems and regulate your feelings. To start, practice the three positions of perception by physically moving around the room. Over time, start shifting them into your mind, so that you always have full access.

Please think of a conflict you frequently encounter with a certain person. For instance, you might often feel your partner doesn't really see you or take you seriously. Or maybe your boss habitually overloads you with many tasks. Or there's that one coworker who's always asking for advice, even though you're up to your eyes in work. Or, or, or . . .

1. Go stand in a certain spot in the room. Channel your shadow child. From this perspective, view the problem

you have with Person XY. Carefully observe how your shadow child feels about the problem, and which beliefs come into play.

2. Shake off your shadow child by patting yourself down or jumping around, then move to a different spot in the room and slip into Person XY's position. View yourself and the situation from their eyes. What are their feelings toward you?

3. Finally, move into a third spot in the room and observe yourself and Person XY like actors on a stage. In other words, occupy your adult-self and analyze the situation from the outside. Think about how you might advise your shadow child.

You must make absolutely certain that the shadow child loses its equal footing with your adult-self. Person XY morphs rapidly into the enemy when viewed from the shadow child's perspective. According to the shadow child, you need to *protect yourself, attack, defend yourself, or flee.*

Here's another example from my practice: Herman, sixty-nine, and Miranda, sixty-five, have been together for a few years. His shadow child's beliefs include, "I can't defend myself," "I have to adjust to you," and "I'm not allowed to be me." Herman's shadow child therefore feels an overwhelming urge to flee and seek freedom. In other words, Herman is a commitment-phobe. In one of our sessions, he told me how he had (once again) gotten upset with Miranda one recent Sunday evening: He'd been planning to come straight home after a short outing with friends. But then his grown son Manny invited him to come over and stay the night, and Herman, who happened to be nearby, impulsively agreed. He called Miranda and told her he'd be coming home a day late. On Monday, his other son, Ben, stopped by to visit his brother, and both young men encouraged their dad to stay just one more night. Herman loved the idea, and he let Miranda know he'd be sleeping over again. At this point, Miranda "started to bitch." Herman was so annoyed that it was all he could do (yet again) not to end things right then and there.

I worked with Herman on the three positions:

- Position 1—The shadow child: "Who is she to boss me around? Can't I do what I want, or do I have to do her bidding now? Is there no room for flexibility? I'm really pissed off!"

- Position 2—Herman steps into Miranda's shoes: "I'm disappointed. I'd been looking forward to seeing him on Sunday evening, and then on Monday evening, and now he's not coming back till Tuesday. He always does whatever he wants. It's like I don't have a say in anything. It's always up to *him* whether he wants to come close or keep his distance."

- Position 3—Grown-up Herman: "Oh, man, it's not Miranda

calling the shots at all—*I'm* the dominant one! I always have to have things my way. When I unexpectedly change my plans, I expect Miranda to just taking it lying down, and even though she does, *I* still feel like the victim. Shit."

By systematically separating these three positions of perception, Herman could view his problem from an entirely new and much more appropriate angle. He spends much of his everyday life occupying the first position, identifying completely with his shadow child. He can't see past the end of his own nose; he thinks only of himself and can't muster any empathy for Miranda. Herman feels like a victim in the first position. In the second and third positions, however, he recognizes his role in the situation and realizes that he's the one demanding too much power—not his girlfriend. This realization changes his feelings and leads him to adopt new modes of behavior. In this case, discussing compromises with Miranda much more often. To help him successfully transfer this exercise into everyday life, Herman and Miranda agreed that he can take a quick "time-out" when things get tense.

Herman is one of those people who protect their shadow child by building a wall between themselves and other people's supposed demands. They withdraw from contact. They can often be found in the first position of perception. People who protect their shadow child by keeping the peace or adjusting to others, meanwhile, often face the opposite problem, namely that they struggle to create boundaries between themselves and others. They get stuck in the second position of perception, meaning they feel and think too much about what other people want and expect from them. These people need to learn to develop a better sense of what they actually want for themselves and what's important to them. In other words, they need to learn to construct better boundaries. This book contains many suggestions for how they might accomplish this.

Discover the Sun Child
Within You

The sun child is an inner emotional state that we all love! But what exactly constitutes the sun child? First, it's the ability to be fully present in the here and now. The sun child loves fun and silliness, and it's curious and spontaneous. It doesn't spend much time thinking about itself, and it likes itself just the way it is. It also doesn't compare itself to other children, because it's focused more on the world around it than on itself. And because it's not constantly watching itself, it doesn't worry about the impression it's making on others. The sun child can laugh out loud, hop, sing, and bound about, enjoying life, but it can also become engrossed in work and learning.

We all possess the potential to experience the fun and joy of a carefree child—by tapping into our sun child, if only occasionally. Think back to how you could laugh out loud and completely lose yourself in play as a kid. Recall the childish curiosity and spirit of adventure you had. Remember the spontaneity and impartiality with which you viewed the world. Consider how rarely you compared yourself to others as a little kid. You should come to realize that the adult norms you uphold today—attractive and unattractive, right and wrong, success and failure—barely registered in your young mind: things just were what they were. Remember the happy moments you had with your family and fun times you had with your playmates.

When we decide it's time to break our old habits and strike a new course, we won't make it very far if we simply vow to stop believing in these old behaviors. We require a vision that we can believe in *instead*. We need a target state of being to orient ourselves toward and cling to, something we can put in place of the old. To that end, we're now going to repeat the exercise you did to discover your shadow child, only this time, you'll be discovering your sun child. This time, we're in search of *supportive beliefs*, and we'll turn our attention to your *strengths*. Furthermore, we will also seek out your personal *values*, which can provide you with support and help you find your way to new attitudes and modes of behavior. And finally, I'll show you ways to build healthier, more sustainable relationships. In short, I will show you alternative behaviors to counter your self-protection strategies. These are known as *self-reflection strategies*.

We want the sun child within you to come into full bloom. The idea here is not to "discover the new you," because most everything about you is already good and just right. Never forget: You're a shining star from day one. We just want to bring positive change to the attitudes and behaviors that sometimes cause you—and, as a result, the people around you—problems. Before we start on the concrete exercises, however, I'd like to share a few thoughts on personal responsibility.

YOU ARE RESPONSIBLE FOR YOUR OWN HAPPINESS

We tend to live in the illusion that other people, events, and circumstances trigger the feelings we have. Just like how Michael, in our opening example, thought Sarah was responsible for the rage he felt because she forgot his chips. Most people think and feel along the same lines as Michael does. If our spouse was in a bad mood this morning, it brings us down. When someone compliments us, it makes us happy, whereas criticism can dampen our spirits or piss us off. We get annoyed by sitting in traffic. We often experience our feelings and moods as something caused by outside forces, whether those are the people around us or incidents we experience. This perception leads us to hold other people or even fate responsible for our problems and moods. We think our unfaithful partner—or our moody boss, menopause, the weather, an unavoidable car repair—is the reason we feel bad. In fact, we are responsible for our own moods and, of course, our own decisions—ultimately, the two are very closely tied. At the end of the day, we determine the attitude and approach we're going to take toward these occurrences. For instance, instead of feeling hurt by our partner's infidelity, we could be pleased that our partner has enjoyed a new erotic experience. We could feel empathy for our volatile boss. Menopause could be welcomed as an exciting time of change. We could simply accept the weather for what it is. Car trouble could be viewed as an opportunity to walk more and/or invest in a better vehicle. Each of these situations could be embraced as a good exercise in patience and composure.

This might all come off as a little absurd and esoteric: who can imagine always being in a good mood, external circumstances be damned? I actually don't believe it's possible, either. It's unlikely there's anyone out there who is totally unaffected by the things other people do or by the personal twists of fate we all encounter, regardless of how much they may have reflected and meditated upon their life. At the same time, we have much more playing room and freedom to shape our own feelings, thoughts, attitudes, and behaviors than we tend to realize.

We can only exercise active influence over our mental state when we accept our responsibility for it. We often fail to realize that we're delegating our responsibilities. I sometimes see this in my clients. Some foster the vague expectation that I'll be the one to solve their problems. They show up on time for every appointment and hope that I'll do something to them that frees them from their woes. But it doesn't work that way. It's impossible to "treat" a patient in psychotherapy the way they can be "treated" medically. When clients expect to undergo psychotherapy passively—if they expect the psychotherapist to do all the work, and they accept this work as a service rendered—they'll never make any progress. Clients who don't accept much responsibility for themselves may, indeed, reach valuable insights during a therapy session, but they fail to implement what they've learned. Other clients, meanwhile, spend the days between sessions working actively on their problems by observing, reflecting, practicing new behaviors, and so on. These folks make speedy progress, whereas the others simply tread water. It's no different with this book: You may just read it and hope that things will somehow improve as a result. Or you can accept responsibility for making changes in your life, and work actively with the exercises presented here.

I'd like you to contemplate the areas in your life in which you are most likely to delegate your responsibilities to others: Where do you think someone else has to change, in order to make you feel better? To what extent do you consider yourself dependent on and governed by external circumstances, or at the mercy of your own moods and attitudes? Your adult-self probably has a few suggestions for ways in which you could take more responsibility for improving a situation or your mood. For instance, adults know that if they're unhappy with their career, it would be better to switch jobs or, if that isn't feasible, to adjust their attitude toward work. They know that if there's something they don't like about their partner, it doesn't make sense to expect their partner to change, and that it's far better to accept their loved one for who they are, or they realize they can improve the quality of their relationship by changing their own behaviors toward their partner. They may also realize when the time has come to split up. Maybe you don't currently have a partner, but hope that one day, someone will come knocking at your door. Warning: That desire is the shadow child speaking. Your inner adult knows that you yourself have to actively engage in the search.

Adults usually know what needs to be done. It's the shadow child that fears change and paralyzes the adult's spirit for action, usually out of fear of failure. Because when I accept responsibility for my actions, I'm also putting myself at risk for failure. This does require a certain frustration tolerance, though, or the ability to endure negative feelings from time to time.

As I explained at the beginning of this book, there are of course certain twists of fate that exist outside the scope of our responsibility and that we can't do much to change: maybe a loved one dies, or we fall very ill. Individuals who live in war zones or conflict areas also have very limited influence over their fate. It's that much harder for them to find their inner bearings to help master their own destiny. Even in the very worst living conditions, however, there are people who manage to attain an inner state that allows them to accept their fate and shape it to a certain degree, even if this means dying.

Since your problems are hopefully less dire than those described above, please try to internalize that you are responsible for your own happiness—100 percent responsible. Don't sit around waiting for others to change or hoping that "something" will happen. Intervene in your own life and change the things you want to change. The following exercises will support you in this move.

* * *

Exercise: Discover Your Positive Beliefs

Now it's time we attended to your sun child. You'll need a new piece of paper (at least 8.5 x 11 inches) and colored pens, pencils, or markers for this and the following exercises.

Please draw the silhouette of a child again. In contrast to your shadow child, this drawing is going to be colorful, nice, and happy. Your sun child will become your target state of being, so the drawing should be very visually appealing. This will motivate you and inspire you to seek out new experiences. Make your drawing as beautiful as if you were trying to win an art contest. Give your sun child a face and other features, and decorate the entire sheet exactly the way you want to (see image inside the front cover).

We're now going to reveal your positive beliefs. We'll do this in two steps: First we'll look at the positive beliefs you adopted from your parents or other caretakers. Then we'll take the core beliefs articulated in your shadow child and turn them into positives.

I. Positive Beliefs from Childhood

If you have a good enough relationship with your parents that you'd like to include them with your sun child, please write "Mom" and "Dad" (or whatever names you used for your parents or caretakers) to the right and left of your sun child's head. This time, think about the positive traits they had. What did they do right? Please write these things down. If you would prefer not to include your parents with your sun child because your relationship with them is or was difficult, you may skip over this part of the exercise. Or list your parents' positive traits on a separate piece of paper and only write down the positive beliefs you adopted from them in your sun child.

Perhaps you also had a loving grandma, a kind neighbor, or an understanding teacher who showed you warmth in childhood. You may also include any of these people with your sun child.

Once you've compiled your parents' or caretakers' positive traits, take a moment to dig deep inside yourself: What are the positive beliefs you gained from these people? Here's a list of examples to help.

> **Positive Beliefs**
>
> I am loved.
>
> I am valuable.
>
> I am adequate.
>
> I am welcome.
>
> I get enough of what I need.
>
> I'm smart.
>
> I'm attractive.
>
> I have a right to happiness.
>
> I'm allowed to make mistakes.
>
> I deserve happiness.
>
> Life is easy.
>
> I'm allowed to be me.
>
> I'm allowed to be a burden sometimes.
>
> I'm allowed to defend myself.
>
> I'm allowed to have my own opinions.
>
> I'm allowed to feel.
>
> I'm allowed to set boundaries.
>
> I can do this.

If you've discovered multiple positive beliefs, please select no more than two and inscribe these in the chest area of your child drawing. As with the negative beliefs, we want to limit ourselves a little here, so that you can work more effectively with these in your daily life.

II. Turning Around Your Core Beliefs

Please refer back to the negative core beliefs you identified on page 73. We are now going to turn these into positives. Beliefs such as "I'm worthless" or "I'm inadequate" are easy enough to reverse: "I'm valuable," "I'm adequate." Some beliefs are a little harder to turn around, however, because we never want to include a negative, such as "not," in our positive beliefs. For instance, if you happen to believe that "I'm responsible for your happiness," the opposite formulation would not read, "I'm *not* responsible for your happiness." The "not" is too tricky for the subconscious to process, because it's difficult to *not* think of something. If I say to you, "Please don't think of a little tabby cat," you automatically start thinking of one. The opposite of "I'm responsible for your happiness" could therefore be "I am allowed to set boundaries," "I can do my own thing," or "My hopes and needs are just as important as yours."

The opposite of a belief like "I'm a burden" would be "I'm allowed to be a burden sometimes." After all, it's unavoidable that we will sometimes be a burden to other people; for example, we might get sick and need help. By the same token, "I'm allowed to make mistakes."

Your positive beliefs should also be formulated in a reasonable way. For some people, it's too great a leap to move from their belief that "I'm ugly" to its opposite, "I'm attractive." I advise these people to tack "enough" on the end: "I'm attractive enough" or "I'm good enough."

To make your beliefs more reasonable, you may also want to narrow them down. If the belief that "I'm important" comes across as exaggerated and unreasonable to you, you could instead write, "I'm important to my children/partner/parents." Phrase your new beliefs in a way that feels good to you.

Please write down your positive core beliefs in your sun child drawing.

* * *

Exercise: Discover Your Strengths and Reserves

In addition to your positive beliefs, it's also important to become aware of your strengths and reserves. *Strengths* are things like character traits and skills that often come in handy, such as your sense of humor, courage, or social competence. Feel free to be generous with yourself here. "Self-praise is no recommendation" is one of the stupidest expressions ever coined. If you have trouble saying something nice about yourself, try to imagine which of your positive traits your friends might praise. Or simply ask them.

Here are some examples to help start you off on discovering your strengths.

Strengths

Athletic	Honest
Attractive	Humorous
Creative	Inquisitive
Disciplined	Intelligent
Educated	Kind
Enterprising	Loyal
Entertaining	Observant
Even-keeled	Reflective
Flexible	Socially competent
Forthcoming	Spirited
Funny	Stable
Generous	Tolerant
Helpful	

Please add your strengths to your sun child drawing (see image inside the front cover).

Your list of *reserves*, meanwhile, will include your sources of strength, or external living conditions that provide you with strength or stability. Here are some examples.

Reserves	
A nice apartment	Kids
Enough money	Music
Family	
Good friends	Nature
Good job	Nice colleagues
Health	Sound relationship
House pet	Travel

Please draw these reserves around the outside of your sun child (see image inside the front cover).

Now that you've determined what your resources are, we'll move on to your values.

HOW HAVING VALUES CAN HELP US

It was long assumed that humans were fundamentally selfish creatures who sought only personal benefit. Recent brain research has disproven this hypothesis: an individual solely inclined toward selfish behavior wouldn't stand much chance at survival. Instead, humans are hardwired to live in groups and cooperate with one another. In his book *Survival of the Nicest: How Altruism Made Us Human and Why It Pays to Get Along*, renowned science writer Stefan Klein argues that altruism can affect our brains in the same way as sex or a bar of chocolate does. When we contribute to society or help a person in need, we love the feeling that our actions are serving higher values. We yearn for meaning in our actions. Conversely, the sense of an action's pointlessness produces depression. Or rather, the sense of all-encompassing pointlessness is a cardinal symptom of depression.

Viktor Frankl, a famed Viennese doctor, developed what is known as logotherapy, which essentially amounts to the therapy of meaning. Frankl argued that people could overcome their existential fears by orienting their actions toward higher values, and thus behaving in a meaningful way. When our actions serve a higher meaning and purpose than our own self-preservation, they allow us to grow beyond ourselves. If I'm afraid to tell my boss my honest opinion because I might then be skipped over for a promotion, I could overcome this fear by remembering that by speaking frankly, I could be shielding a coworker from wrongful blame.

The higher values of justice and moral courage underpinning this consideration can help empower me to overcome my shadow child's fears of loss and denigration.

Values are a fantastic anxiolytic—this is what we call the medications used to combat anxiety. Our everyday actions are governed by values, even if we're unaware of them. We usually first become aware of our values when they're jeopardized. For instance, an attack on justice can unleash tremendous power in us. We can deliberately put these higher values to good use in helping us find strength and inner stability.

Many of the self-protection strategies we use to protect our shadow child cause us to somewhat selfishly focus only on ourselves. We're then so consumed by self-defense that we lose sight of higher values. Here's a little example from everyday life.

Sabrina starts distancing herself from her friend Aisha because she's feeling hurt by a comment Aisha made about her body. Sabrina doesn't want to tell her friend how she feels because she worries it would be a sign of weakness. So instead, she withdraws and breaks off contact with Aisha. At this point, Sabrina could question whether her behavior toward Aisha was really fair. She could orient herself toward the value of fairness, and use this as a way to get past her hang-ups. The same could apply to the value of friendship—after all, they've had a lot of good times, too. Sabrina's retreat doesn't afford Aisha the chance to respond or apologize. Aisha has no idea why Sabrina's been so cold toward her lately. Had Sabrina explained the reason for her behavior, the ensuing conversation could have restored the friends' closeness: the girls could have remained friends, had Sabrina simply opened her mouth. Instead, Sabrina's silent treatment destroys the friendship, because this silent withdrawal also hurts Aisha. Sabrina could have avoided this by deliberately orienting herself toward values, such as fairness, friendship, openness, or moral courage.

At this point, you may be asking why Sabrina should bear all the responsibility, considering that it was Aisha who first insulted her. Yet again, I would point to personal responsibility: Sabrina is the one who feels hurt and is therefore responsible for this feeling. We don't even know if Aisha's comment was actually insulting, or if this whole conflict is based on Sabrina's shadow child misconstruing it as offensive. If Sabrina clings to beliefs such as "I'm ugly," "I'm inadequate," or "I'm so fat," it is quite possible that she misinterpreted Aisha's words as a disparaging critique of her body. Maybe all Aisha said was, "I like the black pants better than the miniskirt," but Sabrina's shadow child heard, "Your legs are too fat for a short skirt!" Sabrina immediately feels hurt without this having been Aisha's intention; it may be that Aisha just didn't like the skirt's cut or pattern.

Supposed insults that actually *aren't* insults happen all the time. The more insecure a person feels, the quicker they are to misconstrue other people's words or actions as containing some kind of personal attack or rejection. This is why it would have been so much more helpful to the friendship if Sabrina had simply piped up. She could have just asked Aisha what she meant by her comment. That's all it would have taken to avoid this misunderstanding. I'd also like to point out that communication can never be 100 percent perfect, just like we and the people around us can never be perfect. There's always a risk that I'll insult a friend without meaning to. Or indeed, I may present an honest criticism that offends my counterpart far more than I anticipated. We can never perfectly predict how others will respond to our words and actions. Even when we take great pains to be respectful and polite, this doesn't guarantee that other people will see it that way, too. We do, however, control the ability to speak frankly whenever appropriate.

If you catch yourself reverting to one of your self-protection strategies, pause for a moment and think very carefully about whether your behavior is actually fair toward the people involved. Whenever your thoughts turn to self-defense, continue to ask yourself whether what you're doing—or even what you're neglecting to do—is *good and proper*. Try to base your behavior less on the question, "How can I best protect myself?" and more on the consideration, "*What is good and proper, and what is meaningful?*" If you elevate this latter question to become your personal guiding principle, you'll be free to grow far beyond your shadow child and its fears. Not only will this help you get by in life, it will also make you a better person.

* * *

Exercise: Define Your Values

I would now like to invite you to uncover your personal values, which can help you overcome the feelings of fear and inferiority plaguing your shadow child. As soon as you start thinking about it, lots of values probably come to mind, such as tolerance, justice, or helpfulness. For this exercise, however, we will limit ourselves to no more than three, for the same reason we limited our number of beliefs earlier—these should be easily retrievable in your everyday life so you can work with them most effectively. It's therefore best to choose those values that function as an antidote to your self-protection strategies. For example, if your self-protection strategies include things like retreat and keeping the peace, you should look for values that empower you to stand up and fight more for yourself (and others). These values could include candor, bravery, moral courage, fairness, responsibility, or propriety.

If you yearn for perfection and try to do everything right all the time, it might be best to embrace "counter values" such as composure, enjoyment of life, trust in God, modesty, or even humility.

If one of your self-protection strategies is an insatiable hunger for power, the values of trust, empathy, and democracy could help counteract your tendencies.

Pick out those values that can help you overcome your shadow child's fears and concerns. I've compiled this list of values for inspiration.

Values

Altruism	Gentleness
Attentiveness	Goodwill
Authenticity	Helpfulness
Bravery	Justice
Candor	Love
Commitment	Loyalty
Compassion	Modesty
Composure	Moral courage
Democracy	Openness
Devotion	Peacefulness
Discipline	Propriety
Education	Reflection
Empathy	Responsibility
Enjoyment of life	Tolerance
Fairness	Transparency
Fidelity	Trust
Friendship	Understanding
Generosity	Wisdom

Please write these words in bright colors above your sun child's head (see image inside the front cover). This placement symbolizes the fact that you've got "a good head on your shoulders," and these values are especially helpful in strengthening your inner adult.

IT COMES DOWN TO MOOD

New beliefs, higher values, and the realization of our strengths and reserves should all help us heal our shadow child and bring our sun child to life. Both acts are closely tied to feelings and moods, because in their own right, all the positive beliefs and superior values in the world don't amount to much if our mood is lousy. Sure, we can make good decisions based on a sense of obligation, but it's so much easier to live life in an "elevated mood," as psychologist Jens Corssen puts it. Corssen plainly describes the way in which our mood can influence the way we think and assess things: When I'm in an elevated mood, I'm friendlier and more amusing, kind, and generous. It makes me feel better, but I'm not the only one—everyone I know benefits from my elevated mood as well. On the other hand, if I'm in a rotten mood, I'll often react irritably and aggressively, or I'll retreat into my shell and seal it up tight.

We're basically always working to keep our mood on an even keel. This has a lot to do with our experience of pleasure: we want to avoid unpleasant experiences and enjoy as much pleasure as possible. In other words, we yearn for happiness. Our paths to happiness can be very different, but there are a few fundamental things that apply to all people. This was already clear to the ancient Greeks, who coined the term *eudaimonia*, which literally means "tied to a good demon." *Eudaimonia* is commonly translated as "happiness" (although experts are not in agreement on the term's most accurate rendering). The ancient Greeks did not view *eudaimonia* as something achieved by means of external factors; instead, it was a state of being that emerged from living life right. This "right" way of living was characterized by self-sufficiency, discipline, and virtue, among other factors. *Eudaimonia* thus stands in opposition to hedonism, or sensuous indulgence. Sensuous experiences unleash an exhilarating, short-term high within us, whereas the "right way of living" leads to a quieter—and therefore more stable—form of happiness. In recognizing this, Plato and his compatriots were as clever then as we are today, because there haven't been any groundbreaking new findings since. Recent brain research simply confirms that, by and large, the Greek philosophers were correct: happiness can be trained and depends largely on our attitudes toward life.

Buddhists don't differ in this view, although their focus is less on achieving happiness, and more on eliminating suffering. Buddhists also have a very clear notion of living right, which they teach in the form of the Noble Eightfold Path. For scientific proof that happiness can be trained, brain researcher Richard Davidson asked the Dalai Lama for permission to research eight monks out of His Holiness's closest circle. The monks were positioned within the narrow tube of a magnetic resonance imaging (MRI) scanner and asked to enter deep relaxation, which they managed to do, despite the loud conditions. Researchers were thus able to observe their brains in a meditative state. The findings came as no surprise to the Dalai Lama: active meditation changes the structure of the brain. The activity observed in the monks' left frontal lobes was much higher than in the control group, comprised of 150 non-Buddhists. This region of the brain—or rather, the activity here—is associated with optimism and good moods. Optimists thus have a more active left frontal cortex than people who usually feel unhappy. This region appears to be responsible for the cheerful disposition and composure enjoyed by well-trained Buddhists and other happy people. The conclusion of this experiment is that happiness is a skill that can be trained like a muscle.

I will be providing you with many more tips and ideas for how to achieve an elevated mood and what goes into the "right way of living." Not only will we use our self-reflection strategies to discover new ways of behaving, we'll also engage our imagination and body memory to install a new feeling—the *sun child feeling.*

USE YOUR IMAGINATION AND BODY MEMORY

Before we produce the sun child feeling in you, I'd like to provide a little more information for your inner adult. As I've already explained, our brain does not differentiate very well between reality and imagination, which is why the latter can be a key component along your path to change. Our brain makes instantaneous associations—both positive and negative—based on images, colors, smells, sounds, and other stimuli. This happens all the time: a view, a melody, or an aroma can trigger a host of images and emotions within you. We're going to take advantage of this mental skill by developing specific positive associations that will help you switch easily into "sun child mode" in your everyday life. Furthermore, we are going to physically anchor the sun child in your body, because the body has significant influence over our moods. Neurobiological studies have shown that our mood not only influences our posture, but our posture also impacts our mood. When we stand up straight, we actually feel more confident than when we slouch along, looking at the ground. Go ahead and try it yourself. You can also stand up, throw your hands in the air, look toward the sky, and try to feel bad. Conversely, you can drop your head and shoulders, stare at the ground, and try to feel really happy. Both will be tricky.

American social psychologist Amy Cuddy has researched the impact our posture can have on our mood. Her studies have shown that both men and women perform significantly better in job interviews when they spend two minutes beforehand striking a "power pose," standing up straight with their legs spread and their hands on their hips. If you'd like to learn more, watch Amy Cuddy's TED Talk, which can be found online.

* * *

Exercise: Anchor the Sun Child Within You

The following exercise is meant to anchor your sun child firmly in your feelings, your mind, and your body. You may also think of the exercise as a *game*, which the sun child greatly prefers.*

It's best to play this game standing up. Place the drawing of your sun child on the floor in front of you. Do a careful scan of your body—how are you feeling? Then focus your inner attention on your chest and belly area, the seat of our emotions.

1. Read your positive beliefs out loud and feel their impact on your body. How does it feel when you say them quietly?
2. Call up a situation in your life in which your positive beliefs are or were already in effect. This could be in time spent with friends, at work, exercising, or on vacation. Or

---

* You can also find this exercise available for download at stefaniestahl.com as the imaginary journey *The Sun Child Meditation.*

maybe when you're listening to music or spending time outdoors. There has to be at least one instance you've experienced in life in which your positive beliefs felt really solid and true.

3. Direct your thoughts toward your reserves. Summon them with all your senses—sight, hearing, smell, taste, touch and feel the power they provide.

4. Turn next to your strengths. Don't just think about them—feel the sensation in your body when you say them quietly to yourself. What feelings do they unleash in you?

5. Move on to your values. Say them out loud, and feel the resonance, the sensations they release in your body. Sense the power or composure they grant you.

6. Feel everything at once—how does your body experience the sun child?

Maintaining this inner state, move around the room to discover your sun child posture. Sense how your entire body feels when you're in this state. Pay close attention to the way your breath moves when you're in this mode. Come up with a small gesture that signifies this sensation. Allow it to emerge from your body. This sign will serve as an anchor in your everyday life, helping you summon this positive state of being whenever you need it. A client of mine spontaneously opened her hand, which suggested a sort of freeform bowl. This relaxed hand pose became her sun child gesture.

Please add these good feelings to the belly area of your sun child drawing.

Add-on: Remain in the positive inner state of the sun child. Then allow an image to emerge from this feeling. You may see the ocean, a beautiful landscape, a playground, or perhaps a cottage in the woods—allow your sun child to present you with this picture. Allow it to surprise you with its gift.

Jot down a cue to recall the image you discovered in your sun child.

THE SUN CHILD IN EVERYDAY LIFE

Your (hopefully very colorful) sun child drawing is the target state of being toward which you can orient yourself. It should provide you with external and—if you spend enough time strengthening it playfully—internal support. We will work on identifying your self-reflection strategies in the next chapter.

Feel free to summon your sun child feeling as often as you want, like we practiced in the previous exercise. If you're in a time crunch, just quickly say your new beliefs and/or values out loud or remind yourself of your strengths and reserves. That beautiful image your sun child produced may be the quickest way to access the feeling. Play around with all these elements. Access the elements that you most need depending on your current situation. It's important that you always take a moment to see what physical effects your beliefs, values, image, and reserves have on you, so that the sun child has a chance to anchor itself in your body.

And of course, don't forget your shadow child because it has a way of sneaking up and surprising you—boo! Then you're back where you started, with your old feelings and beliefs. Your inner adult needs to be on alert, so that you catch yourself as soon as you start reverting to your shadow child. You can then make a clear switch over to your sun child, or comfort your shadow child first. You may also switch directly over to your inner adult to remind yourself that these are old feelings and projections that have nothing to do with your current reality. Revisit the "Catch Yourself and Switch" exercise on page 157.

You should also give your sun child lots of space to develop in your everyday life. It's as easy as just allowing yourself to enjoy life and have more fun in the process. Anything goes, provided it improves your mood and doesn't harm your health or other people. Ask your sun child for ideas—it's bound to have plenty.

It's best to start out your day with a few little games like the following, which won't take more than five minutes.

Laughing is tremendously helpful. Laughing even helps when you don't feel like laughing. It has been found that even fake laughter can have a positive effect on mood. This is the founding principle behind laughter yoga. When I mentioned this in one of my workshops, a participant chimed in, "Laughter damages my depression!" That's exactly right. So take a minute every morning and laugh. Just laugh. You'll be surprised to see your initially fake laughter change to real laughter—maybe even a fit.

Then tack on the following game: Stand with your arms reaching toward the sky, look in the same direction, and say your new beliefs and values out loud. If you like, you can also include your strengths and reserves.

Next, jump around a little and allow old childhood movements to emerge: swing your arms, shake your tush, thumb your nose, etc.

You can also do a little "happy workout" in the morning. Dance to your favorite song or jump on a trampoline. I do the latter every morning (well, almost every morning). Jumping or bouncing movements are associated with good moods in our mind. Trampolines are also ideal workout equipment. They don't cost much, are quick to stow away, and require very little motivation, because you can hop at home.

And of course, you can carry out the imaginary journey *The Sun Child Meditation* at any time (the download is available at stefaniestahl.com).

Your sun child feeling is a wonderful basis for implementing the following self-reflection strategies. Conversely, self-reflection strategies can also help you tap into your sun child in the first place.

On Self-Protection and Self-Reflection Strategies

I n the following sections, I will provide you with techniques for regulating your thoughts and feelings in such a way that you start channeling either your powerful sun child or your rational inner adult as often as possible. The guiding principle will be to dismantle your negative influences and beliefs, with their attending projections and distorted perceptions, and to employ *beneficial* defense mechanisms that we'll refer to as self-reflection strategies. The goal is for you to require far *less* self-defense. In other words, I'd like to help you start liking yourself (even more). The more you embrace who you are, including your shadow child, the less you'll need to hide away from the world. And the more authentically you live your life, the happier you'll be in your relationships. Once you find yourself, you'll have a much easier time with yourself and others—and others will have a much easier time with you.

I will show you how to accept and assert yourself in an appropriate way, in order to find peace with yourself and your shadow child, and to make your sun child smile.

OUR HAPPINESS AND UNHAPPINESS REVOLVE AROUND OUR RELATIONSHIPS

Nearly everything in our lives revolves around our interpersonal relationships. Good relationships make us happy, bad ones unhappy. What good are all the riches in the world if you're lonely? What's the point of great success if you aren't really close to anyone? Profound loneliness is the worst emotional state a person can experience. We have a deep longing to be recognized and to belong to a group. As I've already written, our desire for attachment is existential. This is also why our self-protection strategies are oriented toward our interpersonal relationships: they're intended to help us attain recognition and affection and prevent us from being attacked or rejected.

The entire world operates according to the principle of recognition as a marker of success. Those who desire recognition must be better, more attractive, more powerful, wealthier, or simply "more unique" than everyone else. They may not betray any weakness. As a direct result of this notion, our self-protection strategies mask, at least partially, our authentic self. They help us show our supposedly strong side and hide our weaknesses. We put up the facade we think will make us more lovable, which actually distances us more from others than it does bring us closer. Closeness doesn't come from our being perfect and admired by others for our accomplishments. It also doesn't come from a misguided pursuit of peace, which leads to insincerity. It doesn't come from aggression and attack, from role-playing and disguise, from a desire for power, or from flight and withdrawal. True closeness can only be achieved through *authenticity*, *openness*, and *empathy*.

If you would object at this point and say that you don't even want that much closeness and actually feel best when there's a bit of distance between you and other people, it's a sign that you have fallen back into your self-protection strategy of withdrawal. Even genetically introverted individuals, who really do require less human interaction than extroverts, need to be truly close to at least one person, a person who likes or even loves them the way they *truly* are, in order to be happy. That's ultimately the same thing we're all looking for.

For this reason, the self-reflection strategies are aimed at how to improve your relationships, not how to become more successful. You may very well become more successful through the process of acquiring new self-reflection strategies, but that is no more than a side effect of finding and better asserting yourself. Self-reflection strategies do not serve your *idealized self*—in other words, your wishful thinking—but rather your *actual self.* They help you stand by who you are. Because deep down, we do realize that our actual self will allow us to get closer to others than our idealized self will. After all, we feel best spending time around people who are authentic and stand by their own weaknesses. In the presence of people who appear perfect, we can easily feel inferior and defeated. It's important to remember that, although ideals of perfection can inspire envy, they don't make other people like us: imperfection is endearing.

Most of my clients need help with some kind of relationship problem, whether the issue be with their partner, colleagues, friends, family, or simply everyone. Underlying these relationship problems are always the problems my clients have in their relationship with themselves. This even applies to problems that ostensibly have nothing to do with relationships, such as depression or panic attacks. Relationship problems are often at the heart of these issues, as we saw with Babs in the exercise "Understanding Your Shadow Child" on page 166.

Relationship problems are caused by our shadow child's beliefs and self-protection strategies. This is even the case when the other person is actually more at fault in a difficult relationship—for instance, if they're insincere or scheming—because we still have to consider why we fell for this person. Or why we can't shake them. Or why we constantly get upset with them. Or why we can't distance ourselves from them better. To wit: You can question any relationship based on your role in it. There's also something to be learned from every relationship. We actually learn the most from difficult people, because they push us to our limits. Well-known psychologist Robert Betz refers to them not as archangels, but as "arse angels," an expression I find both funny and fitting. He defines these "button pushers" as angels operating under an inverse sign—instead of helping by doing good, it's their flaws that help us better find ourselves. If one of our self-protection strategies is keeping the peace, an arse angel can help us learn to assert ourselves. Conversely, if we quickly get bent out of shape, interacting with an arse angel can help us practice keeping our cool.

You've probably been there before: some arse angel unfairly judges you or just gets you all wrong. This can cause feelings of rage and helplessness. When someone projects onto me something that I didn't do, say, or intend, it's typically a lost cause. These situations usually can't be solved by means of communication, because the "perpetrator" (the one with the skewed perception) is the one who needs to stop projecting and reflect on what they're doing. If they aren't prepared or able to do this, you're out of luck. These situations are particularly challenging when you're dependent on this individual, whether it's your boss, your wife, or a parent. The more ingrained this person's distorted perception and the less willing they are to question their own views, the less likely you are to reach an agreement with them. Sometimes the only sensible solution is to separate yourself from this person either by breaking off contact or, if that's not possible, creating internal boundaries.

Sometimes, though, *we* are the arse angel for someone else. This makes us both the victim and the perpetrator. We experience what it's like to be treated unfairly, while simultaneously visiting the same injustice upon other people through our own skewed perception. This could be as simple as just ignoring their distress. If we aim to improve our relationships, we have to start with our perception, because it also contains our self-awareness. As soon as we start channeling our shadow child, after all, we lose our equal footing with others. When we feel inferior to other people, they mutate before our eyes into attackers. Or into "idiots," if we're trying to feel superior to them. Perception is the base of our subjective reality, which is why—as with the self-protection strategies—we will first spend some time here.

● ● ●

Exercise: Once More for Good Measure: Catch Yourself and Switch

Learning is all about repetition. I would therefore like to take a moment to remind you of this book's central message: catch yourself whenever you revert to shadow child mode, then release yourself by switching back to your adult reality.

Despite being conscious of our shadow child and its beliefs, we often get caught in its reality. I see this all the time
with my clients: they possess the knowledge they need to
solve their personal problems, but they keep forgetting it. I believe there are three reasons for this:

1. Our inner adult doesn't believe that the matter of the
   shadow child should actually be taken that seriously.
2. We're so thoroughly accustomed to seeing the world
   through the eyes of our childhood influences that it's
   very difficult to believe any other reality.
3. We resist taking responsibility for our feelings and
   thoughts, preferring instead to wait until something happens "out there" that will relieve us.

We tend to identify automatically with our shadow child,
which allows it to go undetected by our consciousness. For
example, Christine, thirty-three, told me about the trouble she
was having subletting her apartment. Her landlord had hired
a real-estate agent to help. The day of the appointment, the
agent showed up half an hour late with fifteen candidates.
Christine was pissed off about the late arrival and the huge
group, which the agent hadn't mentioned. Christine had expected far fewer people. She begrudgingly showed them
around the apartment and then, as soon as the group left,
launched into a fierce argument with the agent. Christine told

this story to illustrate how easily she could go from being in a "good mood" to a "bad mood," and then get caught there. Although Christine had already done a lot of work with her shadow child as part of her therapy, it wasn't clear to her that in this situation, it was the shadow child responding with such rage. By the end of our session, after analyzing the event with regard to her shadow child, Christine was amazed to discover that her shadow child had contributed to her outburst. The fact that the real-estate agent had shown up late, and with fifteen people in tow, had triggered an old conviction of Christine's, namely, "He thinks he can get away with doing that to me." The beliefs "I'm unimportant" and "I'm so small" underlie this conviction. She responded with her self-protection strategies of *attack* and *aggression*. It wasn't the situation that induced these feelings and reactions, but instead Christine's *interpretation* of the situation, which was based on the shadow child's distorted perception. Had she not taken the agent's behavior so personally, she probably would have taken the whole thing in stride.

It's no different for us than it is for Christine: We often don't realize that we're reverting to our old patterns, because they're so familiar to us. It doesn't even occur to us that we could perceive the situation differently. Here's another example from my practice: Leo, twenty-four, told me he had gotten back together with his ex-girlfriend. He wanted to "do everything right" this time. I asked if he had spoken with her about the problems they'd had in the past, which he hadn't. He said he got the feeling that *she* didn't want to, that she just wanted to enjoy the good times with him and forget their past troubles. Leo didn't notice how strongly he was channeling his shadow child. Based on his beliefs, which include "I'm inadequate" and "I can't just be me," one of his most important self-protection strategies is *adjusting*. That is, he tries to meet all the expectations he imagines his girlfriend having. And when he gets the feeling that she doesn't want to talk about their past problems, he goes ahead and avoids doing just that. He perceives his girlfriend from the perspective of a child, trying to be a "good boy" and do "everything right." To that end, he has positioned his inner antennae to receive signals and *intuit* what his girlfriend might expect of him. His fear of rejection and view of his partner come so naturally to him that he often doesn't notice he's channeling his shadow child.

Incidentally, it's usually our feelings that signal the fact that we're channeling our shadow child. Christine could have caught herself descending into rage, just as Leo could have caught himself giving in to his fear of loss.

Always remember that your shadow child can dictate your perception, thinking, and feelings in lots of different situations, even the seemingly banal. And again, if you truly want to solve your problems and grow, it's very important that you accept responsibility for yourself and work *actively* with your new-found knowledge, because this is also the prerequisite for catching yourself whenever you start identifying with your shadow child. Ultimately, you can only change the things you are fully aware of.

DIFFERENTIATE BETWEEN FACT AND INTERPRETATION

If you catch yourself channeling your shadow child and feeling terrible, take a step back, analyze the situation with a little distance, and ask yourself what your *interpretation* of the situation is. In other words, switch over to your adult-self and try very hard to discover the lens through which your shadow child is viewing the world. We're typically reacting to these interpretations, after all, and not the "objective reality." Incidentally, this also applies when the distortion is positive. For instance, we can sugarcoat things in order to protect ourselves from painful realizations. Furthermore, the inner adult and the sun child can also misinterpret a situation. The shadow child's distorted perception, however, is what tends to cause us the most problems, which is why I'd like to examine it more closely.

Many people fail to realize how thoroughly their perception is subjectively colored by the interpretations they're constantly—and unknowingly—making. For example, when Person A thinks, "Why the hell is he smiling at me like that?" she won't usually next examine whether Person B really *is* smiling strangely (read: laughing at her) or he's just a nice guy. A significant part of my work with clients consists of analyzing concrete situations with regard to their subjective interpretations of truth. People who identify closely with their shadow child, and thus have low self-esteem, often demonstrate a strong tendency toward assuming bad intentions of other people. Even when they've been given a compliment, they think that the other person is either manipulating or "fucking with" them. They simply can't believe that another person would view them so much more positively than they do themselves. And even if they do take the compliment, they then live in constant fear of being found out. In other words, they're afraid that the other person might someday discover what they're *really* like. The only thing that doesn't happen is that they question their own negative beliefs and discover that perhaps *they* are the one who is wrong.

Then there are the people we could call "naive," those who view the world and their relationships in a rather glorified light. These individuals have usually developed the self-protection strategy of keeping the peace. They cling to beliefs like "I'll remain a child." They sugarcoat things because they're afraid of facing reality, which might put them in the unpleasant position of actively having to stand up for themselves. People who strive to maintain harmony not only work to avoid conflict, they sometimes don't even perceive it. If you belong to this group of people who are overly gullible and naive, think very carefully about how you would assess the behavior of your conversation partner from a stricter point of view. Try to be very critical. With the help of your inner adult, try to view things as dispassionately as possible. Catch yourself as soon as you start trying to understand the other person and making excuses for them in matters that actually deeply upset you.

* * *

Exercise: Reality Check

The following exercise should help you grasp your interpretations of reality and then change them. Here's an example that you should naturally adapt with your own details.

The concrete situation (trigger) is: My boss alerts me to a mistake.

My shadow child thinks (belief): "I'm inadequate. I have to be perfect. I'm not allowed to make mistakes."

My interpretation: "My boss thinks I'm in over my head and is considering replacing me."

My feeling: "I'm ashamed and scared."

My self-protection strategy: Perfectionism and desire for control. I try even harder, check everything with a fine-tooth comb, and work overtime.

My sun child thinks (positive beliefs): "I'm allowed to make mistakes. I'm adequate."

My interpretation of the situation: "My boss is pleased with my performance, even if I make the occasional mistake."

The adult says (argumentation): "You know a lot about your field. You do regular professional development. Your boss and coworkers make mistakes sometimes, too. Your shadow child is overreacting to this critique."

Feeling: "I will remain calm."

My self-reflection strategy: I'm learning a lot from this mistake, and I will encounter myself and other people, who are also not perfect, with kindness and understanding.

FIND A GOOD BALANCE BETWEEN REFLECTION AND DISTRACTION

We now understand that our interpretation of reality is decisive in how we feel and behave. We still don't always manage to catch ourselves in time to correct our skewed perception and switch from channeling our shadow child to channeling our sun child. We may then get caught in our shadow child's swirling negative feelings. In response, we double down on our self-protection strategies, as if to say: "Bring it on." But this just worsens the problem. If we already tend toward *withdrawal*, we completely disappear into the woodwork; if our self-protection strategy is to be a *jerk*, we become downright aggressive; if we yearn for *perfection*, we start trying even harder, and so on.

In this vicious cycle, we keep feeling worse. We become so entrenched in this mode that we can no longer find a way out.

If you fail to catch yourself in time to correct your perception, before slipping into old patterns, there's another strategy that can help you out of trouble: distraction. Distraction means directing my attention away from my feelings and problems, and toward the world around me. When I concentrate entirely on what's happening out there, or on a task, I stop noticing myself—I forget myself. I feel no pain, whether physical or mental, in this state. Distraction is thus a central tool in psychotherapy for patients suffering chronic pain—he who dances with passion feels no pain in his feet. Fixing our attention elsewhere allows us to forget ourselves, which further allows difficult feelings to subside. Distraction automatically puts you in a better mood, which creates inner distance from your problems.

You've probably experienced the following situation: You're incredibly angry at Person XY, who you feel has misunderstood and treated you unfairly. Your thoughts keep returning to this issue; you obsess over it and get angrier and angrier. Then you become distracted for a while, because you need to focus on your work, for instance. Because you're distracted, your anger retreats into the background, and you calm down. You can now think about your problem with Person XY from a much calmer place. You've gained inner distance. Your interpretation of the situation also changes with this distance. You start seeing the role you played in things. You may even discover you've made a mountain out of a molehill. Or you'll come up with a solution to the problem. The whole thing may no longer appear that important, and you think, "Water under the bridge."

You might be wondering, "So what, then? Should I be carefully observing myself or seeking distraction?" My response: There's a big difference between the two. I might see things clearly enough to allow for personal reflection and, if necessary, to catch myself slipping into a bad state. Or I might become mired in the feelings and thoughts running endlessly—and fruitlessly—through my mind. Immersing myself in my negative feelings doesn't get me anywhere. In sum: It *is* important to observe yourself. However, if you run the risk of getting bogged down by shadow child feelings and beliefs, it's worth distracting yourself first. I can better reflect upon my feelings and problems when I create a little distance.

My advice: Pause from time to time and sense what's going on inside you, then take this awareness back out into the world and pay attention to your conduct. Find a good balance between your self-awareness and the awareness of your surroundings. If you suffer from an acute concern that constantly demands your attention, I would suggest you take half an hour every day to delve into this problem in writing. This lets your inner adult know that, whatever happens, everything is on paper, so you can spend the rest of the day tending to other matters.

To stop yourself from coming back to your problem repeatedly over the course of the day, you can put a rubber band on your wrist. Whenever you catch yourself thinking about your problem, simply snap the rubber band on your arm to redirect your attention back to the task at hand.

BE HONEST WITH YOURSELF

As we've discussed, self-acceptance doesn't mean that I think everything about me is great. It means accepting myself with my strengths and weaknesses. I'm also not talking about self-love. "Love" is such a big word. It's enough simply to enjoy living, because it means we like the fact that we exist.

The degree to which I can accept myself depends on the extent of my self-awareness. After all, I can only accept the things I'm aware of. If I only accept the things I like about myself, though, I'll need to block out or suppress the other parts. Many people will therefore swerve a little around their self-awareness: they focus on weaknesses that are relatively harmless, or even nonexistent. Weaknesses that would actually be worth examining more closely, meanwhile, are pushed into the furthest corners of their consciousness. I once had a drop-dead gorgeous client who honestly spent our entire first hour-long session sobbing because she thought she was so ugly. This is, of course, an extreme example of distorted perception, but it illustrates a point: this client's weakness certainly wasn't her appearance, but rather her pronounced tendency toward hysteria, or a totally excessive reaction. And just like my client, who was so misguided in her concerns, we all experience this to varying degrees.

When I close my eyes out of fear of painful realizations, I may be protecting myself from these images, but I'm not developing at all. For instance, if I don't admit to myself that I run away from big decisions because I'm afraid of failure, I just end up treading water. If I don't admit that I'm incredibly envious of a certain person, I will never be able to resolve this feeling in a healthy way. If I don't admit where the limits of my capabilities lie, I'll never be satisfied with my achievements.

I encourage you to be as honest with yourself as possible. It can help to ask a good friend for their opinion, because it can be hard to view ourselves objectively. Honest self-perception can be incredibly cathartic, because it reduces our fear. At the moment I admit that my skills are insufficient for realizing my dreams, for example, I no longer need to fear this admission. I can relax and acknowledge, "That's just how it is." And I can then create more realistic plans for the future.

There are usually vague fears of certain truths at play within us. As long as we run away from this truth, from this recognition, the fear will remain in place, and we won't develop any further. If I pause for a moment and admit to myself that, "That's just how it is," then the fear can dissolve and perhaps make way for a certain grief. It can create room for new things. Maybe I provide new direction for my desires, such as focusing on a different occupation, one that's a better fit. Or I just accept that my talents won't take me to amazing heights, but are certainly good enough to achieve satisfactory results. I might decide to compensate for what I'm lacking in talent by working harder. Whatever the case, it's only after realistic self-assessment that I can regulate my goals and actions in such a way that I end up much happier than when I was running in the opposite direction out of fear of self-awareness.

When working with our weaknesses, the worst conclusion we can reach is that of guilt. Feelings of guilt are almost unbearable. It can be incredibly cathartic, however, to admit our guilt to ourselves. Simply to say, "Yeah, that wasn't cool," "Yes, that was my fault," or "True, I would never do it that way again." I have to take responsibility for my own actions before I can find justice for my victims. I have to admit to my mistake before apologizing to the people it affected. More often than not, these are the people closest to us. If you discover that you're sorry about certain things you've said, done, or even neglected to do, you should consider apologizing to the people your actions impacted. Many adult children are incredibly relieved when their parents finally concede that, "We're sorry. We were overwhelmed back then and would do things differently today." Our shadow child often has permanent scarring because our parents never held themselves accountable for their mistakes, and instead justified themselves or denied any wrongdoing. Perhaps you, too, desperately wish that one or both of your parents would finally just apologize for the things that went wrong in your childhood.

If you have grown children and realize, after honest self-critique, that you made some of your own mistakes as a parent, apologize to them. This apology can be a new beginning in your relationship. If your children are still small, closely examine the ways in which your shadow child might influence your parenting and try to be as self-aware and reflective as possible in your actions.

If you retrospectively realize you did wrong by a friend or coworker, apologize for it, even if it was years ago. Because conversely, there have probably been situations where you were the victim—where someone did wrong by you. Imagine if that person finally apologized to you. How amazing that would feel!

* * *

Exercise: Say Yes to Reality

This exercise is actually an inner stance I would encourage you to try. It is drawn from Buddhist meditation practices, which I'll admit aren't exactly in my wheelhouse. I do know that a cornerstone of these meditative exercises is to affirm and accept things as they are. I think that we can adopt this simple idea in our lives without having to immerse ourselves in Buddhist philosophy. The notion of saying yes is mentally easy to grasp. As we've seen, resisting painful insights can cause chronic, subliminal pain in us. Resisting fear requires more energy than accepting it. This is the case with all of our negative feelings: grief, helplessness, rage, shame—they dissipate most quickly when I accept them.

When I talk about fear, I'm talking about the shadow child. When we accept our shadow child—and thus, all our fears, feelings of inferiority or shame, sadness, and helplessness—it starts to feel understood and can gradually begin to quiet down. It can be enough simply to say "That's just how it is" a few times a day. Maybe you have to go to the dentist, or you're thinking about a conflict with a friend, or you're stuck in traffic, or the kids are annoying you, or you missed the train, etc.: keep saying to yourself, "That's just how it is." It works best if you combine the sentence with your breath, inhaling deeply, exhaling, and thinking, "That's just how it is." Keep this up, and you'll see how calming and cathartic it is.

Feelings are always a transient state. We know this from our feelings of happiness. Whenever we're really happy, we know from the get-go that it won't last forever. Negative feelings such as lovesickness or fear, however, can sometimes feel like they'll never go away.

Think back to the exercise I described in the section "How to Snap Out of It" (page 75): Concentrate on the physical manifestation of this difficult feeling. If you're sad, for instance, focus on what's happening in your body. Maybe there's a lump in your throat, or pressure in your chest. Concentrate on this feeling alone, and block out all the images in your mind associated with your sadness. If you're sad because your girlfriend dumped you, block all the mental images you have of her and sense only the physical feelings of sadness in your body. Stick with it. You'll discover that it soon dissipates. You can use the same technique with any other difficult emotion. This exercise is derived from the Sedona Method, a pragmatic approach to dealing with feelings developed by Lester Levenson.

PRACTICE GOODWILL

The inadequacy that our shadow child often feels not only affects our own well-being, but also influences our attitude and behavior toward other people. From the perspective of the shadow child, other people can quickly transform into enemies. Insecure people often live their lives on the defensive. They're constantly afraid of being the underdog, vulnerable to attack. Those who are busy defending themselves, however, cannot simultaneously muster sympathy for their attacker. As a result, they're unable to feel goodwill toward the person they consider their superior. I can only muster goodwill toward people I see as being on my level. However, if I feel inferior, I won't only be hard on myself, but on everyone around me as well. I may admire certain things about the people I consider superior, and think that I'm only being harsh on myself, but to be perfectly honest, that isn't really the case. Schadenfreude—taking pleasure in others' misfortunes—and envy are all-too-human traits and tend to be aimed at people we perceive as being above us. Our shadow child can be incredibly petty and wary of others. That's why it's best for my community that I channel my sun child or inner adult as much as possible. It improves my mood and as a result, I perceive those around me more favorably. Perception and mood exist in perpetual interplay. When I'm in a good mood and encounter other people with kindness, they'll feel good in my company. It creates a positive dynamic. It's much more relaxing to view other people favorably than to wait anxiously for the next attack. The tenser and more stressed out I feel, on the other hand, the more likely I am to project these feelings onto other people, thus creating a negative dynamic.

It's easier to feel goodwill toward other people when I'm channeling my sun child. Conversely, if I'm being petty and aggressive with myself, it will be all the more difficult to act with generosity toward others. That's why it's so important to look after myself and accept responsibility for my own well-being. You can accomplish this by showing understanding for your shadow child and comforting it, as we practiced in the section "Consoling the Shadow Child" on page 153. At the same time, train yourself in activating your sun child. See to it that your mood improves. View it as your duty to have as much fun in life as you can. I'll be going into this in greater detail in the section "Enjoy Your Life" on page 231.

Goodwill is also an inner stance I can choose to adopt. Many people who identify with their shadow child practically insist upon meeting others with distrust. Suspicion and distrust are among their self-protection strategies, and because they identify so closely with their shadow child, they also truly believe the things they perceive and think, namely: the world and everyone in it are selfish and evil. To avoid any misunderstanding: I don't mean to suggest that humans are fundamentally good. A naive image of humanity is as problematic as habitual distrust. However, by embracing a fundamentally distrustful view, without a hint of goodwill, we help make the world just a little bit worse. Furthermore, the distrustful, pessimistic stance that all humans are essentially selfish has no basis in science, as I described in the section "How Having Values Can Help Us" on page 186. As a reminder: Modern brain research has shown that we humans are programmed to cooperate, and that giving makes us happy. Thus there are rational arguments to be made in favor of taking a benevolent stance toward others.

If you catch yourself judging a friend, colleague, relative, or partner in a petty, negative way, take a deliberate step back and try to analyze the situation from a more generous, favorable perspective. In the side note "In a Bad Mood? It Could Be

Genetic" on page 49. I explained that unfortunately, it's in our genes to better remember and place more emphasis on negative experiences. As a reminder: One negative interaction can displace one hundred positive experiences. So, before you come to the conclusion that Person XY is acting on base ulterior motives, use the help of your adult-self to examine whether this is *really* the case, and reflect on how many good things you've experienced with this person. Thoroughly consider whether your interpretation of the situation is valid. We're often far too quick to suspect others of wicked intentions, even when it's a longtime friend. A forgotten birthday, a small verbal jab, or the "wrong" reaction can disappoint some people so deeply that they come to doubt the very basis of their friendship. By adopting a more generous attitude, we concede that, just like us, other people

- primarily prefer doing good things to doing bad;
- will still sometimes make mistakes;
- can be forgetful, even if it's their best friend's birthday;
- might experience anxiety, which causes them to be somewhat dishonest at times;
- can fail to calculate the exact consequences of their actions;
- simply aren't in the mood from time to time;
- sometimes act without thinking;

- are sometimes in a bad mood; and
- all too often channel their shadow child.

Bear in mind that difficult people often have a deeply troubled shadow child.

Human relationships aren't perfect. We all make mistakes, so try to be as generous as possible with your own shortcomings and those of others. Aggression and pettiness are primarily harmful to yourself—they depress your mood and strain your interpersonal relationships. Speaking of mood, humor can help us build relationships with greater levity and goodwill. On that note: I'm not flawed—I'm quirky!

PRAISE YOUR NEIGHBOR AS YOU WOULD YOURSELF

Goodwill also means that I praise or compliment others from time to time. This is hard for a lot of people when they're channeling their shadow child. Caught in this inner state, they tend instead toward envy, which allows very little room for praise, if any at all.

Some people are also too shy to pay a compliment. It's as embarrassing for them to pay a compliment as it is to take one. They're accustomed to this from childhood. Many people are taught growing up that "silence is praise enough." Others believe, perhaps self-righteously, that they simply have very high standards, both toward others and themselves, which is why they rarely pay compliments.

Whatever the reason people struggle to praise or honestly compliment others, I encourage them to practice generosity in this regard. If you recognize this in your own life, just try to be more giving toward yourself and others. Pat yourself on the back for the things you do well, praise yourself for your appearance and possessions, and applaud your good deeds. Start your day with self-praise—which happens to come highly recommended. Praise yourself as often as you can. This will improve your mood and reduce any feelings of envy you may experience. You could also try taking the route of gratitude: Be thankful for everything that's going well in your life. And be grateful for everything that you have, and that you all too often take for granted. Try to focus your attention on the goodness in yourself and your life. All the griping about your own supposed weaknesses and deficits leads to ingratitude. Self-praise and gratitude help you build up a sense of appreciation, which you can then start sharing.

Praise your spouse, children, coworkers, boss, friends, and people on the street. Americans are quite open with their praise for strangers: it's not unusual to hear "I love your dress!" from a cashier at the supermarket. I like this nice, open manner. By comparison, we Germans are rather reserved and uptight, although things have been improving in recent years. (And I don't want to hear the line, "Americans are so superficial." An employee in a German supermarket doesn't exactly show profound spiritual depth just because they don't praise others for their outfits.)

We all want to be acknowledged. Rather than passively waiting around to be praised, start actively paying compliments to others. And speaking of "paying"—your generosity should extend from your appreciation of others to your finances. Stinginess is a terrible quality that far too many people exhibit. If you are someone who balks at showing generosity, examine your beliefs very closely and analyze your stinginess as the self-protection strategy it is. Believe me, your greed doesn't make you happy, nor does it contribute any security to your life. On the contrary: the more you give, the more you'll receive. You'll see how much your mood and relationships improve once you start treating other people with generosity in all its forms.

JUST GOOD IS GOOD ENOUGH

As we've been learning, most people expend a tremendous amount of energy muzzling their shadow child, with its negative beliefs. Many hope that by striving for perfection, they will silence the child. Allow me to reiterate: These beliefs are negative illusions. They are wrong, and at most, they are an expression of some of your parents' shortcomings. You are also making mistakes, though, in your choice of self-protection strategies. While yearning for perfection, you become overly concerned with the question of what impression you're making on others, and spend too little time questioning what actually makes sense.

To strengthen your inner adult, you can pose a number of self-critical questions: Why do you want to be perfect? Is that really why, or is it because you want to limit your vulnerability? Or do you want to be admired? Please take a step back and view your behavior from the outside. Who—other than you—considers it important that you produce perfect work, look perfect, or act as the perfect host? How much of this is ultimately just you? Imagine all the extra energy and time you would gain if you eased up on your quest for perfection and did "just" a *good* job on things. What would you do with all that time? Is there any chance you're afraid of boredom or painful memories? Or are you suppressing serious problems by escaping into your work? Lots of people try to outrun their problems by staying as busy as they can. As soon as peace and quiet settle in, their fears and concerns come a-knocking.

Strengthen your adult-self by considering the problems you might be fleeing. Ask whether your self-protection strategies might not be causing you more problems than they're helping you solve. Perfectionists tend to be stressed out a lot, which puts strain on them as well as on their relationships. Remember that because of the high expectations you have for yourself, you may also be overly strict with those around you.

Furthermore, your ambition is curtailing your enjoyment of life. Keep in mind that you're at greater risk for burnout than people who are more relaxed in their approach.

Then ask who would benefit if you invested less time in your perfection. Your family? Friends? An aid organization? Or maybe even just you, because you would start having more joy and fun in your life?

Try to relativize your perfectionism by asking what the point is. Take your shadow child by the hand and repeatedly remind it, lovingly and patiently, that it is good enough just as it is, and that it's allowed to make mistakes. Then strengthen your inner adult by seeing your frightening imagined scenarios through to the end: Would you *really* lose your job if you worked less? If so, consider whether the stress is worth it, or if it might be possible or beneficial to make a career change.

Consider whether your relationships really *would* be better if you were the perfect friend or lover. Besides, what does "perfect" even mean here? Then run through your standards of measurement. Instead of being the most gorgeous, the best, or the most awesome, wouldn't it be much more "perfect" if you were really honest and open instead? What would be perfect for those around you is knowing where they stand with you and that they can rely on you. It would be great if you didn't always base your actions on your likelihood of success, but more on the question of what you think is right. What if, instead of trying to be perfect, you just tried to be yourself? If you tried to channel your sun child as much as possible? If you tried to be more relaxed?

Remind your adult-self of two things:

1. The world through the eyes of your shadow child is a projection, a negatively distorted reality.
2. There are so many more meaningful things to do than to be perfect. For instance, being a decent person and enjoying life.

ENJOY YOUR LIFE

Many people, ensnared in their shadow child's self-protection strategies, don't dare enjoy their life. They simply indulge far too rarely. They overextend themselves at work and in other obligations and believe that they're not allowed to enjoy themselves until everything has been finished. But there's always something they have to do next. Their shadow child feels a sort of fundamental guilt, namely the guilt of "not being good enough." They're convinced that they don't deserve enjoyment in life, or they make their own existence so onerous that there isn't any room left for joy. They feel guilty whenever they aren't working. People whose self-protection strategies include power-hungriness or perfectionism have an especially hard time shutting off from time to time.

From the perspective of our inner adult, however, there

isn't any rational argument to be made in favor of not enjoying life. "What use is a miserable life?" my father would always say, a quote I love. Please remember that enjoyment in life puts you in a good mood. It brings out your sun child. Start to see it as your obligation to do what it takes to feel good and enjoy your life. This does require strong time management—because enjoyment takes time. Chronic procrastinators are often as unable to enjoy themselves as control freaks, because they, too, suffer a guilty conscience. The difference between the two is that procrastinators *should* feel remorse, because they avoid necessary tasks, whereas control freaks feel the need to perform even inconsequential tasks perfectly, which leads to the guilt they carry. You can find more tips for taking care of business in the exercise "Seven Steps Against Procrastination" on page 302.

Good food and good wine can make us really happy. The same can be said for a walk outdoors, music, or good sex. Enjoyment is of course linked to personal preferences. Denying yourself enjoyment, however, is not an acceptable solution. Please allow yourself to enjoy life as often as you can.

Some people are so out of practice, they no longer know how to enjoy things. They habitually overextend themselves and are usually stressed and ill-tempered. Others feel like they need a "good" reason to take a break, such as a headache. This upsets the sun child, but no one asked its input—if they did, it would surely have lots of fun suggestions. You would just need to lend it your ear for once. Given the chance to develop, your sun child would know exactly what it takes to be happy.

If you have the tendency to spread yourself too thin, say something along these lines to your shadow child: "Hey, sweetheart, you know we don't have to run ourselves ragged to feel valuable. You are valuable, even if you take time to rest occasionally. You need to take breaks in order to restore your energy. If we overextend ourselves to the breaking point, no one really benefits. We're allowed to take free time and relax. We're allowed to enjoy life and have a good time. Then, once we've recharged our batteries, we can really hit the ground running."

Fun and enjoyment are also linked to beauty. Look around you and consider whether there are enough things in your workplace or apartment that please the eye. Find some nice things to look at, things that make you happy. If you're using this book to work on internal renovations, do the same to make external changes to your surroundings. It can be something small, like a pretty flower on your desk. Scents can also make us happy: I always carry a little bottle of rose oil with me, and whenever I need a quick pick-me-up, I dab some onto my wrists like perfume. Accept responsibility for feeling good. Look after yourself.

For several years, psychosomatic clinics have offered therapeutic programs to teach people how to enjoy again. Enjoyment has a lot to do with consciousness. After all, I need to engage my five senses to experience enjoyment. If I'm unob-servant, meanwhile, I really can't enjoy things. If I wolf down my food, for instance, I can't even tell what I'm ingesting. In these therapy sessions, participants' senses are honed. Partici-pants are instructed to describe precisely what they perceive when eating a piece of chocolate or looking at a rose. This teaches them conscious enjoyment. You can easily introduce this "enjoyment therapy" into your everyday life. There are just two things you need to do:

1. Arrange for enjoyment by doing things that feel good more often.
2. Be entirely present in the here and now with your atten-tion and all five senses.

Another good way to increase your awareness of beauty and enjoyment is to go on walks and pay close attention to the beauty you see around you. Imagine you have a camera—or actually bring one with you—and look for beautiful moments to photograph. Keep your attention trained on your external surroundings. It's really not easy, but it's hugely relaxing for your mind, because it distracts you from yourself. I practice this a lot when I go for walks, because I'm one of those people who can quickly slip into their inner thoughts and lose touch with what's going on around me. The sight of beautiful flowers and natural surroundings can make me very happy, though.

DON'T BE GOOD, KID—BE AUTHENTIC

People whose self-protection strategy is keeping the peace want to do right by everyone around them. They learned this as children, as a way to gain their parents' attention, or at least to avoid their punishment. They have a very hard time creating boundaries between themselves and other people's wishes and needs, and they feel responsible for others' well-being. If their companion is in a bad mood, peacekeepers will feel guilty and wonder what they did wrong, or what they could do to cheer this person up. Because of the constant attention they pay to the other person's real or imagined needs, they neglect their own desires. This can't last forever, of course, because ultimately, they'll want to be given their own due. Because they so rarely express their wishes—and even then, they're barely audible—these individuals constantly have the feeling of coming up short. Although they also hold this against themselves, they primarily blame the people around them, who they perceive as dominant, which I described in the section "Self-Protection Strategy: Keeping the Peace and Overadjustment" (page 101). Just as they're constantly trying to sense what other people want, peacekeepers expect others to do the same for them. When this doesn't happen, they very quickly become offended.

People who strive for peace and harmony accept too little responsibility for themselves, because they're constantly concerned with the well-being of others. They want to do everything right and not hurt anyone. If they're up-front about it, though, they aren't really doing this for the other people—it's for their shadow child, which fears rejection. After all, if they were more open about their needs, they might rub someone the wrong way. To avoid this, they adjust to what they think are other people's expectations and hope that the others will "thank" them by returning the favor and also anticipating their needs.

If the paragraph above sounds familiar, the first step is to remind yourself, with the help of your inner adult, that you are trapped in your childhood mind-set. In order to please your parents, you tried to adjust as best you could, perhaps because they were very strict or cold. They actually may have been very loving, but tried to maintain peace and avoid conflict themselves. This did not provide you with a strong model for self-assertion.

In any case, you were very dependent on your parents as a child. Explain kindly to your shadow child that those times are past and that you are now responsible for your happiness. You have a lot to learn when it comes to taking care of yourself. Accept responsibility for your well-being. Say what you want and don't want. In no way does this make you selfish. On the contrary: When you advocate for yourself and your desires, then others will know where they stand with you, and you can negotiate things fairly. This is far better than pouting when your friend fails to intuit your wishes. Don't forget that your withdrawn demeanor requires other people to rack *your brain* if they want to know what you're thinking and what you want. This becomes a lot of work for them over time. Besides that, they never really know where they stand with you. It would be a big relief to them if you were more open and authentic about yourself. Taking responsibility for yourself means they no longer have to. They no longer have to ask, repeatedly and fretfully, if it's *really* okay with you to do something this way and not that way.

It's just as important that you defend your opinions. If you aim to do right by everybody, you actually aren't doing right by *any*body. You're not really answering for anything, and ultimately, no one can depend on you. You don't need to be everyone's darling—it's more important that you grow a spine and swim against the current every now and then, when it's a question of values and other important things. Bear in mind that moral courage, propriety, and justice are always more important than your worries about slipping down the social ladder. There might be some people who don't like you that much when you express your opinion, but they don't like you that much when you don't express it, either. As I've said, they don't know where they stand with you, and they might even think you're a little boring. To that end, just relax: You'll never be able to please everybody. So develop your own opinions and benchmarks. Keep reminding yourself that it's not about winning points with other people—it's about acting according to your values.

You might be thinking, "That won't amount to anything!" People who avoid conflict love saying this. First of all, opening your mouth can help a lot more than you might think. Second, you should never base your actions solely on the likelihood of success. For instance, if you tell a good friend that you found a certain behavior of his really offensive, you're giving both him and your friendship another chance. It's a chance to have a conversation to clear things up and restore your closeness. You have then done everything within the realm of your responsibility to improve the relationship. That's what it all comes down to. How the other person responds no longer falls upon you.

Perhaps your problem is that you don't really know what you want or think. Are you so conditioned to watching out for others that you can no longer connect to your inner life? If so, then listen very carefully to what happens inside when you ask, "What do I feel?" and "What is my opinion?" You can also practice standing up for your opinions by staging an imaginary debate and arguing your stance with a make-believe opponent. Practice this in real life as well. Catch yourself whenever you notice you're reflexively starting to stifle your opinions and/or needs in an effort to be liked. Then channel your sun child and start to speak. You'll be amazed at how much easier life becomes when you behave more openly and honestly. Your relationships will become much less complicated. It is only once you are truly authentic and accept responsibility for yourself that *real* harmony and nearness can emerge.

LEARN TO DEAL WITH CONFLICT AND SHAPE YOUR RELATIONSHIPS

People who protect their shadow child by adjusting to others and trying to keep the peace are governed more by circumstance and chance than by setting goals or clearing their path of roadblocks. In order to set goals, they would need a clear vision, which they usually don't have, because their whole life has been oriented toward other people, instead of themselves. Another reason for their passive approach to life and relationships is their fear of conflict. They live under the shadow child's impression that they simply have to submit to relationships rather than exercising influence over them. They don't act—they *react*. This habitual adjustment takes a toll on healthy self-assertion. These people are often so accustomed to adjusting to those around them that it doesn't even *occur* to them that they could express their opinions or needs. It never fails to amaze me how little inclination some people have to put up a fight. As I described in the section "Self-Protection Strategy: Keeping the Peace and Overadjustment" on page 101, individuals who fear conflict often assert themselves in passive resistance, which can lead to withdrawal, flight, or breaking ties.

There's another reason these people are so reluctant to speak for themselves: they're uncertain whether they have a *right* to their opinion and desires. They're not particularly adept at argumentation. Because they view other people as superior, they default to granting them greater rights and competence. It is therefore absolutely critical that they work on feeling *secure in their own standpoint.*

Many people don't dare argue; they're afraid of defeat, so they keep their mouth shut. They think in categories such as "win/lose" and "superior/inferior." They go on the defensive to supposedly protect their shadow child. Fear of being the underdog extends beyond the peacekeepers to those we refer to as "jerks," whose self-protection strategy is aggression and attack. They try (in vain) to get the best of the situation, typically overshooting their mark.

If you shy away from conflict, view this fact from the point of view of your adult-self. Remind yourself that it's not about winning or losing. If your conversation partner makes a better case on a given topic, it doesn't mean you're inferior. You simply say, "You're right," and preserve your confidence. Adopt the inner attitude that it's a question of *the topic at hand*, and not your performance. Most important, use your adult reason to remind yourself that it's entirely okay to say what you want and have your own opinions. In most cases, the conversation will not escalate into conflict. In most cases, no one will even take it the wrong way if you say no, but more on that later. First, I'd like to introduce a few rules of conflict resolution.

* * *

Exercise: Practicing Conflict Management

For this exercise, please think of a simmering conflict you're having with someone, either because you've already argued or because you haven't yet dared tell this person how you feel.

1. Deliberately channel your sun child. Call upon your new beliefs as well as your strengths and values, and take note of how good these make you feel. In other words, try to get into as good a mood as possible. If this doesn't really work, switch over to your adult-self and try to view the situation with as little emotion as you can.

2. Remind yourself that the person you're facing in this conflict has a shadow child of their own, and that you're on equal footing with them. Try to muster a sense of goodwill toward them.

3. Being honest with yourself, analyze your relationship with this person. Do you feel inferior to them? Superior? Are you envious of them at times? Or do you look down on them? Assess whether there's anything within you that would distort your perception of them. Try very

carefully to recognize the part you play in the situation. It can be helpful to run through a reality check, as we did on page 213, and/or "The Three Positions of Perception" exercise from page 169.

4. Maintaining your inner state, whether sun child or adult-self, consider the arguments supporting your stance. It's best to write these down. Try to imagine the other person's arguments. Feel free to ask other people for help with this: What arguments do they come up with, either for your side or the other person's? Once you've gathered all the arguments, assess whether the person you're fighting with might actually be right. If so, tell them, and your conflict will be resolved. If not, move on to step 5.

5. Arrange a meeting with this person to speak about your concerns. Do not wait for it to "happen when it happens." Present your concerns in a friendly manner, and refer to the arguments you have developed here.

6. *Listen very carefully* to what this person has to say on the subject. Respond to their arguments, and take them seriously. Remind yourself that it's not about winning and losing, but the matter at hand. If the other person has better arguments that unexpectedly change your mind, simply tell them that they're right. In this case, you maintain your dignity and solve your problem. If the person doesn't have better arguments, you can simply stick to your position or, better yet, work out a compromise.

You don't need to adhere to this sequence exactly. It is merely an example of how you can prepare yourself for a necessary discussion or dispute. I'll demonstrate how to do this in everyday life with a concrete example below.

Please remember that you can approach anything—even tricky problems—in a positive mood, channeling your sun child. Nothing is lost by being presented in a friendly way. If you approach the other person with goodwill and respect, there's nothing you can't discuss. And never forget: Admitting that the other person is right, if they are indeed right, is a sign of both confidence *and* likability. Conversely, if you obstinately insist upon your own poor arguments, you appear neither confident nor very nice. *Arguments, goodwill, and insight are the pillars of every agreement.*

Here's an example of a successful conflict resolution: Lara and George are coworkers. Lara feels that George interrupts her too often in meetings, but because she's shy and fears conflict, she doesn't put up a fight. He recently cut her off yet again, and Lara realized she had to do something. She was really pissed off.

1. To calm down a little first, Lara looks around for distraction. She decides to work on a task that requires a lot of concentration. This gives her enough distance to start channeling her inner adult (she could have switched over to her sun child as well, but her anger was too extreme).

2. After calming down some, Lara analyzes her own role in this situation: She admits that she's been letting George get away with this behavior, because she hasn't put up a fight, thus taking too little responsibility for herself. She discovers that she's been tapping into her shadow child whenever George interrupts her, and that she is then paralyzed by her beliefs that "I'm not smart enough," "I'm not good enough," and "I have to be nice and well-behaved." Lara realizes that because of her own beliefs, she has been assuming that George doesn't take her seriously or respect her.

3. She has now calmed down to the point that she can start actively channeling her sun child. In this state, Lara tries to analyze George's behavior from a place of generosity. It dawns on her that she isn't the only person George interrupts; he does this to other colleagues as well. She reminds herself that aside from the interruptions, he's actually a nice coworker. Lara ultimately realizes that George doesn't behave this way out of disrespect toward her, but because he's impulsive and temperamental. She thus no longer views his behavior as a reflection of herself and her supposed inferiority, but as something entirely on his end. This is a new and positive interpretation of reality.

4. These insights reestablish Lara's equal footing with George. She now starts to wonder whether she even has

a right to call him out on his behavior, or whether doing so would be petty and overly critical. After all, he probably means no harm. She could also just be a bit gutsier and insist on finishing what she's saying. Finally, though, she decides it would be nicer to talk about the situation *together* with George.

5. Lara then thinks through the pros and cons of having a word with her coworker: "Pros: It would be good to discuss things with George, because only then will I know how he sees things. It's only fair to let him know that his behavior rubs people the wrong way—and probably not just me. The sooner I can make this point, the calmer and more composed I'll be. Cons: George might take my critique the wrong way. He might not even accept that his behavior isn't okay. But I have concrete examples to support my claim—if George denies these, then he has a problem receiving criticism. If that's the case, it's not my fault, and it was worth a try."

6. Lara decides to speak with George. The next day, she asks if he'd like to take his lunch break with her, an invitation he happily accepts. As they're eating, Lara amiably describes to George how it makes her feel when he interrupts her during meetings. George immediately acknowledges her critique, apologizes, and vows to improve. He says that he's aware of this weakness, and that he can be overly impulsive sometimes, but that he certainly

does not intend to be mean or disrespectful. He prom-
ises to be more disciplined. Furthermore, they agree that
if George goes over the top again, Lara will simply take
the floor back.

Thanks to George's immediate understanding, there was no
need to argue. Because Lara addressed the problem, George
was given the opportunity to respond and confirm her suspicion that when he interrupted people, it was because of his
own overexuberance, not out of disrespect. The conversation
consequently brought the two coworkers closer together.

The potential conflict that could have arisen between
Lara and George was quickly resolved, thanks to Lara's consideration and self-reflection, along with George's open self-
criticism. When at least one conversation partner refuses to
reflect upon themselves and remains locked into their self-
protection strategies, the discussion will probably fail. The
following section examines one such case.

RECOGNIZE WHEN IT'S TIME TO LET GO

There are unfortunately also situations in which good arguments won't get you anywhere, even if the other person's aren't
any better. You face a losing battle when your conversation
partner forces their distorted perception and projections onto
you. That's why it's so important to practice argumentation, to

help you discern which of you is actually the crazy one. Commonly, the root of the problem is that you don't know whether you're accurately assessing the situation. In other words, you need a clear view of things, to avoid getting entangled with an "arse angel" for no reason. In these situations, talking doesn't help. All that helps are outer—or at least inner—boundaries. Without question, you can be in an elevated mood and still accomplish this. On that note, I would like to quote Jens Corssen again, who suggested initiating a separation as follows: "You are a shining star, but you're behaving unfav'rably, and because you are sadly clinging to this behavior, I have to part with you."

However, even friendly boundaries are only successful when you accurately assess the situation—in other words, when you recognize that arguing is pointless. You're probably wondering how to accomplish this. One essential criterion is how willing your counterpart is to respond to your arguments. Are they really listening to you? Do you feel understood? And very important: How *concrete* are their arguments? If the person you're arguing with criticizes you, then they need to be prepared to attach this criticism to something concrete you have done. For instance, if they accuse you of always being dominant, they must substantiate this accusation with concrete examples. Of course, it could be that they're projecting a certain dominance onto you because of their own feelings of inferiority. Don't take it personally. If your conversation partner isn't prepared to support their criticism with tangible, reasonable examples, then they are in the wrong—if only for the fact that they owe you real reasons for criticizing you. On the other hand, if they're actually right, you probably already know it. In this case, there's only one way forward: apologize and vow to improve! The dumbest thing you can do is deny valid criticism. Your conversation partner could come to the conclusion that it's pointless trying to talk to you, because you don't take criticism well. Keep reminding yourself: Mistakes aren't a disgrace. The disgrace is denying them.

Your conversation partner may, however, cite examples for their criticism that are not based in fact, but in their interpretation of reality. It is critically important that you distinguish here between interpretation and fact. I would like to illustrate this point, using the example of Lara and George again: It's a *fact* that George repeatedly interrupted and spoke over Lara. This is a concrete behavior observable by third parties. Lara's *interpretation* could have been that George is a disrespectful macho man. Indeed, this was her initial assessment. Had Lara not been as reflective as she was, she could easily have accused George of just that—either loud and clear, in which case he would have had the opportunity to respond. Or she could have bottled her anger, without giving George that chance. In the second instance, Lara would have distanced herself from George and potentially vented her anger to other coworkers. In the worst-case scenario, Lara's misinterpretation and fear of confrontation could have led to widespread workplace bullying, with George, the supposed "dominant offender," as its target.

If your counterpart is unable to present sound arguments that extend beyond assumptions—that is, beyond their subjective interpretation of perceived reality—then there's something rotten going on. Especially if and when they insist on their incorrect stance. For instance, if George assured Lara that he meant no disrespect, but that he was just a "blabbermouth" sometimes, Lara would do well to believe him, especially if she was unable to produce any additional facts to substantiate her interpretation. Always remain as wary of your own interpretations as you are of other people's.

Furthermore, when it comes to relationship issues, contrary to widespread belief, it does not necessarily take two to tango. Metaphorically speaking, if a mentally sound person is sitting in a boat with an extreme narcissist, that boat is bound to capsize. It's psychological law. The healthy person cannot save the relationship—they will succumb to the narcissist's skewed perception. The possibility for communication in these situations is often greatly overestimated by psychological laypeople: if your communication partner is trapped in their shadow child's distorted perception, not even the most measured words can help. The best protection against powermongers is to avoid them entirely—or start a revolution.

You can be certain that the other person is in the wrong if

they pigeonhole you based not on facts, but on their "gut feeling," and then insist on the veracity of this image of you. You can try to show them they're wrong, but please don't do it too often. Beware of falling into an *orgy of justifications*. At some point, you must draw the line, because again, this is the exact losing battle caused by the other person's obstinacy and inability to self-reflect. They're protecting their shadow child by means of power hunger, meaning they always have to be right and can't allow themselves to get so close to you that they actually start listening. This person's empathy is limited—at least in this situation—because of this self-protection strategy. And with that, we have arrived at one of the most valuable self-reflection strategies in interpersonal togetherness: the ability to empathize.

PRACTICE EMPATHY

Empathy is the ability to feel for other people. If, however, I'm too busy thinking of myself and my own problems, I am quick to lose sight of other people's needs. Everyone's been there: if you are currently plagued by physical or emotional ailments, it can be hard to concentrate on anything else. Our entire organism yearns for the pain to stop. As a result, we are best equipped to feel empathy for others when our own needs have been addressed to the point that they no longer demand our full attention. Some couples will thus find themselves in a permanent bind. For instance, a woman may expect her husband to satisfy her needs for attention and understanding before she can muster empathy for him. In fighting to be understood herself, the wife loses her sense of empathy for her spouse. Incidentally, this is another good argument for the inner adult to look after itself: the more control I take over my own happiness, the more relaxed I can be in approaching my partner and other people.

It is especially difficult to feel empathy for a potential or actual attacker. Nature designed it that way: if I have to defend my life, I can't feel concern for my enemy. The issue in our civil society is just that our supposed attacker often *isn't* one. Or rather, that this person is our partner. As you know by now, when we get trapped in a state of fear and insecurity—in other words, when channeling our shadow child—we often imagine enemies where there aren't any. Empathy is thus most accessible when I'm feeling secure. When feeling self-assured, I can open up to others and experience empathy for them.

As I described in the side note "Problem Dodgers and Non-Feelers" on page 78, there's another reason some people struggle to feel empathy for others: they have a poor connection to their own feelings. This often applies to men, who are more likely to get trapped in patterns of rational thinking. Constructive discussions with less empathetic individuals are still possible, however, provided they manage to approach others with goodwill and interest. Because intellectually, these people can still understand what their conversation partner is saying. Generous, albeit less empathetic individuals can sometimes be very helpful to talk to, because of their rational approach to things.

Far more problematic than an overly logical, but attentive, conversation partner is the first case described, namely someone who channels their shadow child and considers themselves the victim of a supposed oppressor. This skewed perception can lead to a sort of mercilessness in which the supposed victim feels only pity for themselves.

It can be especially crazy to see this at play within couples. Here's a case from my own practice: Linda and Jonathan had been married for almost twenty years when they scheduled a consultation with me. They were seeking advice on sexual issues they were having. Jonathan had had no interest in sleeping with Linda for years, which deeply upset her. Even early on, their sex life had been punctuated by long dry spells on Jonathan's end. During our psychotherapy sessions, I discovered that as soon as we broached the subject, Jonathan immediately and completely reverted to his shadow child. When the conversation turned to his low sex drive, within milliseconds, Jonathan recast Linda as the enemy and became rigid and dismissive. The beliefs underlying his hostile, distorted perception of Linda included, "I'm responsible for your happiness," "It's my fault," and "I have to fulfill your expectations." His shadow child saw Linda as a superior force. He projected his cold, disdainful mother onto Linda. Accordingly, Jonathan went to great lengths to make Linda happy. This included the fact that he often said yes when he really meant no. His self-protection strategies included keeping the peace, adjusting to others, and role-play. As a result, he accepted too little responsibility for his own well-being in the relationship. His needs came up short.

As is so often the case, Jonathan held these unconscious grievances against his wife—whom he viewed as superior—much more than against himself. He passive-aggressively punished Linda for this by withdrawing and withholding sex. His underlying (unconscious) defensive stance might read, "At least in the bedroom, I can do what I want." In other words, Jonathan's shadow child took a stand against fulfilling Linda's sexual expectations (on top of all her other expectations). Sleeping with his wife would have been just another obligation. Precisely because he felt so responsible for his wife's well-being, Jonathan denied her the fulfillment of her wishes—a common paradox. Whenever Linda tried to get close to him, he didn't see her need for intimacy; instead, he perceived her as demanding, intrusive, and possessive. Jonathan lacked the empathy needed to access Linda's needs for intimacy and acceptance, the same reason he was unable to sense that his sexual refusal was insulting and hurtful to her. Nor did he realize that his wife was in a powerless position: No matter what she did, there was no approaching him. He was merciless in that regard. It wasn't until Jonathan changed his perspective and stopped seeing himself as the victim that he could finally feel empathy for Linda. This allowed a new closeness between them to emerge, with positive consequences for their sex life.

If you discover that you're overly wedded to your own take on a problem you're having with another person, try to gain some distance from your feelings and tap into your adult-self. Become an outside observer—imagine yourself on a stage, for instance (or run through the exercise "The Three Positions of Perception" on page 169). With this inner distance, try to understand the dynamics of your problem. What is going on between you two? Problems often center on concerns of acknowledgment (you both feel underappreciated by the other) and justness (you both feel unfairly treated by the other), and as a result, the problem becomes about ill will. Make a conscious effort to feel beyond your own pain to what the other person is experiencing. Put yourself in their shoes and feel what they're experiencing with you. What concerns, fears, or wounds does your behavior trigger in them? Try to understand their shadow child. This act of empathetic insight may provide a new level of access to your problem.

Please keep in mind that it's easy to change the things that lie within your control. This isn't the case with changing people. If you spot an opportunity to approach someone by means of empathy, take it. Don't wait for them to make the first move. Approaching others is a sign of strength, not weakness.

JUST LISTEN

One of the greatest virtues is the ability to truly listen to others. Listening is the bridge to empathy. But many people struggle with this. Their thoughts easily wander, usually back to themselves. What's more, I get the impression that things are going rapidly downhill for our listening culture. In my parents' generation, folks could easily manage conversations with up to twelve people around the dinner table. Today, this usually falls apart at about four, because people interject their thoughts, start side conversations, or simply take out their phones.

Good listening can be practiced by actively *doing* it. It's about more than a conversational technique—it's an inner *attitude*. Namely, being *truly* interested in what the other person has to say. In order to be receptive to them, the first step is to put aside your own concerns and thoughts for the time being. Imagine stowing them away in a vault and locking the door. Since you hold the key, you know that you can open the vault again at any time. Your worries and personal thoughts will be kept safe there. Remember that constantly thinking about yourself is usually an attempt to gain control over your problems. But when your problems are safely locked in the vault during the time you need for listening, you can relax and turn all your attention to your conversation partner. Focusing on another person can make you forget yourself, which can be very healing.

Most people will respond to certain cues—whether mental or verbal—by turning back in on themselves. Rule #1: Always keep your focus on the other person. If self-centered thoughts start to creep in, send them straight back to the vault and redirect your attention toward your conversation partner. Many people are quick to start talking about themselves: For instance, you want to tell a friend about your trip to Italy, but within moments, they take the floor and start reveling in memories of *their* last vacation. Pretty annoying, right? (Just a little tip: Even in minor moments like this, you can intervene in your life and take back the floor and the conversational focus. Simply say, "Would you please just listen for a minute? I wanted to tell you something!")

The second step is to repeat what's been said in your own words. This confirms that you've correctly understood what the other person has told you. This process is called *reformulation*— you are formulating what was said in your own words. Here's an example:

Anita: "Recently, ugh, I don't know . . . I've been feeling completely run down. Work every morning, then the kids with all their demands in the evening. And I don't have anyone to help me. Then my boss puts all this pressure on me. I'm usually so on edge that I blow up at the kids and anyone who gets in my way. I need a vacation so bad."

Ben: "Sounds like you're totally exhausted."

Anita: "Yeah, absolutely."

This reformulation makes Anita feel she's been heard, and it encourages her to keep talking. It also provides an opening for a direct explanation, should Ben have misunderstood anything. This probably seems pretty banal, but it's small things like this that often cause our understanding to founder. Always remember that we tend to *interpret* what's been said, which can quickly lead us astray, especially when we're listening with the ears of our shadow child. If Ben weren't a good friend or co-worker of Anita's, for instance, but was instead her partner, he might be prone to taking her words as a personal critique. What he "hears" might be "I'm not doing enough for her."

If all went well, Ben-the-boyfriend would then check his interpretation by nicely asking Anita, "You think there's more I could do to help?" This question would then give Anita the chance to confirm or correct Ben's interpretation. Most important, however, she would realize that Ben had felt indirectly criticized by her words, and she could respond accordingly. But if things didn't go so well, Ben-the-boyfriend would keep his interpretation to himself and directly launch a counterattack, listing all the things *he* had on *his* plate. This could easily make Anita feel criticized and overlooked, culminating in a fight.

Reformulation is simple and difficult at the same time. Simple, because you can vastly improve the quality of your communication using this method, which is easy enough to understand. Difficult, because it isn't easy to distill everything that's been said. Here's another example:

> **Jan:** "So I recently got a message from Sandra asking who did the catering for my birthday party. I asked her if she was planning a party, and she said no. Then today, Peter asks me if I'm invited to Sandra's summer party, too!"
>
> **Richard:** "You must feel really dissed."
>
> **Jan:** "Exactly!"

Reformulations that hit the nail on the head can really help the speaker along. Until Richard reformulated things, Jan hadn't fully realized just how "dissed" Sandra's behavior had made her feel. However, even reformulations that don't totally hit the mark can be useful to your conversation partner. Because even if the reformulation is inaccurate, the speaker needs to consider briefly whether that really was what they wanted to say, which can help them clarify their thoughts and feelings. In both cases, the speaker feels as though their friend really wants to understand what they're talking about.

It can be very helpful to start by saying, "Am I understanding you correctly . . . ?" For example, "Am I understanding you correctly that Thing XY is seriously bugging you?" After hearing this lead-in, the speaker feels invited to correct their listening partner if they feel misunderstood. Furthermore, it strengthens their sense that the other person really feels for them.

There have probably been many times when you felt utterly misunderstood because your conversation partner wouldn't budge from their view of things. You may have done whatever you could to explain your side, to no avail. Reformulations—especially those that begin with "Am I understanding you correctly . . . ?"—represent the exact opposite of such tedious verbal power struggles.

Incidentally, reformulation is a method used in *client-centered psychotherapy*, which was founded by American psychotherapist Carl Rogers. I am trained in this approach myself, and a core part of my work is in reformulation. You can practice reformulation in every conversation you have. To keep within the confines of this book, I've only touched upon the topic here. There are many guides available if you would like to expand your understanding of "active listening."

SET HEALTHY BOUNDARIES

People who keep the peace and adjust to the needs of others are often incredibly helpful. If they demonstrate signs of "helper syndrome," however, they'll extend themselves far beyond their own emotional and physical bounds, in order to rescue others from plight. Some even force their help upon others. They need this other person (who is, themselves, supposedly in need of help) to stabilize their feelings of self-worth. In so doing, they neglect their own needs. Instead of taking care of themselves, they prefer taking care of others. They hope to receive gratitude and appreciation in return. Their shadow child thinks they have to make themselves useful if they want to earn people's recognition.

If you've ever flown on an airplane before, you know that safety precautions and emergency procedures are always outlined before takeoff. Should there be a change in cabin pressure, oxygen masks will drop from the ceiling. And who should you put the mask on first? That's right: yourself! Because you need to be getting enough air yourself in order to be able to help others. You cannot take responsibility for other people if you aren't taking enough care of yourself.

If you suffer from helper syndrome yourself, remind your shadow child that it doesn't need to sacrifice itself for others in order to increase its worth. Your inner adult should take on the responsibility for your feelings and needs by actively seeing to

it that they are fulfilled. Don't wait around for other people—
or more accurately, those people receiving your help—to take
care of you. It's important that you start paying more attention to yourself. That doesn't mean you should become incon-
siderate and selfish. After all, your willingness to help is also
a positive attribute. Hang on to it. The more self-confident you
become, however, the easier time you'll have distinguishing
between who really needs your help, and who doesn't.

Work on finding a better balance between self-care and
care for others. The first step is admitting to yourself that you
have a right to self-care and self-assertion. Lots of insecure people doubt their personal "bill of rights." Take your shadow child
onto your lap and tell it you're really happy it's there. Explain that
it doesn't need to fight to be welcomed. Keep explaining that
you're both big now, and that the world out there isn't like it was
with Mommy and Daddy. Promise that from now on, your inner
adult is going to be in charge, and will take better care of it.

You probably don't know what it is you want, exactly, because you've always paid more attention to the wishes of others than to your own. Practice taking note of your own needs,
as I outlined in the section "What Can I Do If I Don't Feel
Very Much?" on page 81. Become the focus of your own perception. Listen to your body. People who have a deeply insecure shadow child are often accustomed to feeling very little
about themselves, including physically. I'll be sharing some
concrete exercises for the body in the section after next.

When interacting with others, take careful note of how you feel around them. Stifle the impulse to guess at their desires and needs. And, most important, open your damn mouth and say what you want, and what you don't want! Accept responsibility for yourself. Don't expect your conversation partner to read your mind.

If you feel trapped in a relationship in which you are dependent on a person who refuses to change, no matter how much you try to help, you must remind yourself that things only *seem* to be about them. In fact, your shadow child is projecting its need for acknowledgment onto this person! Your shadow child is using this person to prove its worth. Remember that your worth is not dictated by your partner's behavior. Escape the mirrored self-esteem you've been conditioned to accept, which I described on page 33. If you've been vying for your partner's approval for as long as you can remember, the time has come to abandon the hope that they will ever change, and start to appreciate and approve of yourself. Think about ways in which you can find your own fulfillment independent of your relationship. It is very important that you take your happiness into your own hands. Find a new hobby, or get back into an old one. Meet up with friends more often. Seek out professional development programs. Treat yourself to wellness. Do whatever it takes to become happier and more content, and don't wait around for your partner to change.

It's also possible that you have a passive fear of commitment. This would mean that you habitually choose partners who don't really open up to you; or, if they *do*, you quickly lose interest in them. Work on this. Redirect your energy and attention to yourself. This will create a healthy distance between yourself and your unhappy relationship, allowing you to work on the one person you have direct influence over. Basically, all your inner adult needs to do is direct its overactive helpfulness toward the shadow child. The better you take care of yourself, the more your batteries can recharge. In the end, this will also allow you to participate much more fully in the world around you.

SIDE NOTE: THE SHADOW CHILD AND BURNING OUT

Burnout can occur whenever an individual puts incredible sustained effort into a task, but fails to find success. They might fail to gain the appreciation of their boss or coworkers, and/or their efforts might not yield their desired results. People working in social professions are especially susceptible to burnout. For instance, medical caregivers tend to work on extremely tight schedules, but despite their best efforts, they always have the feeling that their patients are coming up short. People in other professions—managers, athletes, civil servants, office workers, and students—frequently report feelings of exhaustion as well. Burnout is increasingly being diagnosed as such, an indication that doctors and psychologists have become more attuned to its symptoms. It also shows, however, that pressure in the workplace has increased exponentially in recent decades. In many fields, employees are being pushed to produce more in less time.

Burnout is a form of depression brought about by extreme exhaustion. The term "burnout" has become established as a more socially acceptable designation: it can be easier for people to talk about burning out than about being depressed. They may fear that others hear the word "depression" and think "mental illness" or "personal failure." They therefore prefer the sound of "burnout."

In addition to difficult working conditions, personal proclivities may pave the way for burnout. People who suffer burnout are often perfectionists. Because they don't want to do their work just well, but *perfectly*, it's easy for them to become obsessed with details. Candidates for burnout are often workaholics. A typical symptom of workaholism is the inability to distinguish between important and unimportant things: at a certain point, it becomes as critical to lay out their clothes for the next day as it is to prepare the year-end report. They simply want to have control over everything. Remember that perfectionism and power hungriness basically go hand in hand.

In addition to having a combination of difficult working conditions and characteristic perfectionism, people who experience burnout exhibit two further qualities that predestine them for this brand of misery: first, they don't know their own limits, and second, they're bad at creating boundaries between themselves and the demands of their surroundings.

The shadow child within burnout victims has latched on to adjustment as a self-protection strategy. This means that the shadow child works so hard to do everything right, in an effort to receive praise and recognition—or at least to avoid censure—that by the end, it no longer has any feeling left over for itself. For this reason, a big part of therapy for those suffering burnout is to regain a sense of self. They are given exercises that promote self-awareness. As I've repeatedly emphasized, people whose methods of self-protection center on adjustment focus so much on the needs of others that they lose sight of their own needs. It is thus critical that the burnout victim learn to recognize their personal needs. The next exercise, "Allowing Your Feelings to Dissolve," can help with this.

The second step is for clients to take responsibility for their own needs, which they do by learning to assert and take better care of themselves. After all, the burnout wouldn't have come to pass had they refused certain demands leading up to it. You have as much right to say no in the workplace as you do at home. We'll examine this more closely in the section "Learn to Say No" on page 269.

If you would like to avoid burnout, you must practice self-awareness, develop a sense of your own limits, and learn to assert yourself. Lots of the exercises in this book can help you with this. Additionally, using your critical, adult mind, assess your working conditions. Question what you're really working your ass off for. Question whether it's *really* necessary. Question whether you might actually prefer changing jobs. It is critical that you create some distance between your shadow child (with its attending self-protection strategies) and yourself, and that you then view your situation from the outside. As you know, I'm a big fan of argumentation, so try to reframe the entire situation in terms of rational arguments. Paint yourself a realistic image of your work performance, and take a closer look at both your strengths and weaknesses. Employing your arguments, evaluate the point at which your performance limit has been attained. It can be very helpful to speak with coworkers, or even your boss, about your performance and objective demands at work. Carefully examine your own inner motives: What is driving you in this way? Is it really just external demands, or is your shadow child, with all its fears of failure and rejection, involved in some way? It's likely the latter.

After completing your rational analysis, take your shadow child in your lap and explain things along these lines: "Oh, poor sweetie. You always work so hard to do a good job and get everything right. Pretty soon, though, you're going to reach the point where you can't do anything at all. And look, it's okay if you just do something *well*. You don't need to prove anything to yourself. Things with Mommy and Daddy weren't always easy. You always tried so hard to make them proud and happy. But that's over now. We're big now and can take care of ourselves. And you are good enough! You're absolutely fine, exactly the way you are. It's okay to rest and let yourself take a break. Our worth has nothing to do with our work performance. We're also going to start saying no more, and only take on as much work as we can manage. I, your inner adult, am going to take responsibility for you from now on. In order to protect you from feeling overwhelmed, I'm going to stop accepting every task that comes my way. It's no good to anyone if we fall apart at some point. And just think, you poor thing, we're even allowed to rest before we reach that point. It's actually our job to make sure we're doing okay. Because that's the only way we'll be able to survive for our company and our family."

The following exercise should help you gain a greater sense of yourself. It is not intended exclusively for candidates for burnout, but for anyone who would like to become more aware of their body.

* * *

Exercise: Allowing Your Feelings to Dissolve

You can do this exercise standing, sitting, or lying down. It has been borrowed and modified from the Sedona Method, developed by Lester Levenson.

1. Close your eyes, and notice how you're feeling. Sense how your body feels. Pay attention to your breath. Direct

your inner attention to every last corner of your body. Simply take note of how your body feels. Sense where there's tension. Send your attention to the parts of your body that feel tight or cramped. Send your breath to these spots, allowing them to relax.

2. Think of a problem you would like to let go of. Sense how it makes your body feel. Do you feel pressure? Or a tugging? Is your heart pounding? Your breath catching? Take note of the feeling. Welcome it.

3. Intensify the feeling of this problem by imagining yourself ratcheting up your self-protection strategies. For instance, if you tend toward perfectionism, imagine trying to do everything even better and more perfectly. If your way of dealing with a problem is to retreat and repress, then imagine yourself withdrawing entirely, no longer capable of doing anything. If your idea of solving problems is through aggression and attack, then imagine becoming even more belligerent. Sense what happens in your body as you intensify your self-protection strategies. Does the tension in your chest increase? Does the tugging in your belly worsen? Do you start to sweat?

4. Breathe deeply into this feeling, and allow the mental images of your problem to disappear. Banish them. Pay attention only to your physical feelings. Breathe into the parts of your body that house these feelings, until they disappear. Take note of how this feels. Be atten-

tive to your body in everyday life—notice whenever your shadow child or this problem begins to manifest physically. Breathe into the problem, and allow the feelings to dissolve on the bodily level. You can then consciously switch over to your sun child, as we practiced in the exercise "Anchor the Sun Child Within You" on page 197.

LEARN TO SAY NO

One of the biggest problems facing people whose shadow child sees itself as inadequate is difficulty saying no. They're afraid of disappointing other people. They want to do right by everyone. Their shadow child's fear of rejection dictates their behavior. Their shadow child believes that if it does everything right, it might be good enough after all. As with all other adjustment strategies, the problem here is that what's right and what's wrong isn't assessed by means of the inner adult's balanced arguments, but by *what other people think*.

I would like to come back to the projection that's often at play in these cases: I project the disappointment I think people will feel if I say no onto these very same people. In order to prevent this dismay, I obediently rush to say yes. For instance, when a volunteer is needed for some task, whether in my sports club, at a community meeting, or at my kids' school, I dutifully raise my hand. And I do this even though I'm already spread way too thin. All this effort just to comfort my poor shadow child. The problem is that in the shadow child's reality, a "no" can lead to sanctions or even expulsion from society. But that isn't true. Clients who learn to say no more often, will tell me in amazement that other people don't seem to have any problem with this, nor with their not volunteering every single time. Furthermore, they tell me that since they've started taking on more responsibility for their own wishes, their energy levels have been much higher, just because they occasionally turn down a request. This then leads—surprise, surprise—to an improved mood. And as we've learned, being in a good mood is the best prerequisite for being a good person. When your mood and energy levels are good, you can also feel good doing someone a favor. I would like to reiterate that this is not about becoming more selfish; instead, it's about treating yourself better. Lots of people who are trapped in patterns of self-defense are usually stressed out, exhausted, and in a bad mood. This means they don't feel good saying yes *or* no.

If you're often uncertain about whether you have the right to turn down a request, or rather, if you're afraid that the person asking will be disappointed if you do, then get your inner adult to help you come up with some rational arguments. Instead of always worrying if you have the right to say no, think about this: What right does the other person have to be angry or disappointed if you do? So when your neighbor asks you to bring a pie to the barbecue, but you don't have time or any interest in baking, just tell her that, and ask if there's anything else you can contribute. What right does she have to hold that against you, and what arguments would support that? And what right does your partner have to be upset when you start standing up for your desires and needs? Remember that when we agree to do a favor against our will, we usually end up holding it against the other person, which damages the relationship more than if we'd just said no in the first place. Remember that you can also negotiate a compromise. After all, you're big now and can help shape your own relationships.

TRUST IN YOURSELF AND IN LIFE

Control is our response to fear. And because fear is a fundamental part of life, we all exhibit a great need to control ourselves and our surroundings. The desire for control is much stronger in some people who need a lot more of it to feel safe. Their shadow child feels powerless and at the mercy of others. It's terrified of letting go and feeling trust, because it has no trust in itself. If this resonates with you, then have your inner adult ask, "What's the worst that could happen?" We don't usually think this question all the way through, but will instead act on our shadow child's vague fears. What would really happen if you relaxed a little and trusted more in yourself and in the ebb and flow of life? Take the scenario that causes you such fear and see it through to the very end. Push yourself to the limits of your imagination, and keep asking yourself: "And then?" Look your worst nightmare in the eye and ask yourself whether it's *really* that bad, or whether it might not still have the potential to be worked into something else.

Once you've thought and felt through this dreadful scenario, deliberately create distance between yourself and your fearful shadow child. Channeling your inner adult, explain the following to your shadow child: "Oh, you poor kid. You're still so hurt from the past. Things weren't easy with Mommy and Daddy—you didn't have any chance to speak your mind, and you always felt you weren't good enough. But we're big now, and everything you're so afraid of is really unlikely. We can find help whenever we need it now. Not to mention, we can defend ourselves. We've also learned a lot and can do a lot. And always remember: we're free now, and we're allowed to have our own free will. What's going to happen to us? Worst case, we go on welfare, which is still better off than a lot of people on earth. Worst case, [name of partner] breaks up with us, but we'd survive that, too."

Always remember that your fears are projections. Most of the things we fear will never happen. Or, if they do, we'll figure out a way to deal with them. People who are plagued with fears must learn not to believe everything their shadow child thinks. Think about how often your fears have misled you. How often did things work out far better than you had feared? Or far worse? If the fearful voice in your mind—in other words, your shadow child—were a consultant for your company, you would have fired it (effective immediately!) a long time ago, for all of its inaccurate forecasts. The point is, there's a lot we can't control in life, and our predictions both good and bad—are frequently off the mark. For this reason, keep reminding yourself that the big things are out of your control, anyway. The more you cramp up, trying to hold on to and control things, the tougher it will be for you and the people around you.

People who yearn for control over things as a means of self-defense often have an overblown sense of obligation. In its most extreme form, this can lead to pathological compulsive behaviors or thoughts. In less dire cases, individuals will follow extremely disciplined routines that cause them significant suffering. Relinquishing control is challenging because it requires these people do the one thing they struggle with most: trust.

But how do we learn to trust? If I'm not terribly religious and don't put my fate in God's hands, then what I need is a good sense of trust in myself as I turn to face this life. The more trust I have in myself, the more certain I'll feel in my ability to survive and accept defeat. My desire for control is intended to protect me from the negative feelings that crop up when I make a mistake. If I want to let go more, then I've got to learn how to tolerate these feelings. The frustration tolerance we've spoken about so much comes back into play here. I have to believe in my ability to handle frustration, in order to clear my mind. This makes room for the idea that actually, I'll probably be successful—or at least, nothing bad is likely to happen.

Fear is a result of the equation *probability of occurrence* x *catastrophic potential.* People who are afraid of flying, for instance, know that the probability of crashing is very low, but because the catastrophic potential of such an occurrence is so great, the idea of flying terrifies them. When people are afraid of failure, they consider both the probability of occurrence *and* the catastrophic potential to be very high. First, their shadow child thinks they'll probably fail, and second, that they won't survive the fallout. Both levers can be adjusted to provide relief: your shadow child needs to be consoled and supported in the face of its negative beliefs. As always, the key is to dismantle your own projections. We've already learned how to do this. Comfort your shadow child and explain the way the world works. Keep strengthening your sun child and inner adult. As always, your inner adult is strengthened by means of argumentation.

An important argument your inner adult could make here is not to take itself so seriously. Whenever we give in to our fears of failure, we're usually taking ourselves too seriously. If your adult-self would just create a little bit of distance from your shadow child—thus occupying the third position of perception—you would see that, in global terms, your own failure is utterly meaningless. The problem is that our fears make us think we're the center of the universe. This might sound paradoxical, considering that our fears make us feel humble and guarded. This is true, to a certain point, but the fears we feel about ourselves are by nature egocentric, because we're constantly focused only on ourselves. For this reason, it can be relaxing and therapeutic to habitually relativize our own importance as well as that of any potential failures.

Is your desire for control so extreme, however, that you also crave power? Do you always have to have the upper hand, always have to be right? Please question the motives behind your behavior: What's *really* going on? Get it into your head that it's not always about winning and losing, but that other values—such as understanding, cooperation, friendship, and respect—are often far more important. Speaking of respect, this could be a sore spot for you. Examine carefully whether you might not demand more respect from others than you show them in return. You may insist others treat you with the utmost respect, but you don't realize that in doing this, you're forcing them to adjust to your expectations. Make no mistake: your desire for power forces other people to conform to you, and you owe them the same respect you demand for yourself. Be mindful of staying on *equal footing* with the people around you. As soon as you tap into your shadow child, you lose this equal footing, insisting that you're right and trying to gain the upper hand. Using your adult mind, tell yourself that you're big now, and that the world out there is not the same as "Mommy and Daddy." You are free, and no one has power over you. Your power struggles cause far more problems with other people than they solve. You're grown up and independent now, which is why you can surrender some of your control. At the end of the day, you would actually love to just let things happen as they happen, and to feel trust.

If you would like to practice letting go and trusting, it could be helpful to learn some relaxation and meditation techniques. Be patient if these exercises take a while to figure out: the demands you put on yourself sometimes make you irritable when you aren't an instant pro at something new. Exercises in "mindful release" have their roots in Buddhist meditation. If this interests you, I would recommend reading a book on the subject or downloading an app to help you explore these practices.

REGULATE YOUR FEELINGS

When we get caught up with our shadow child, it isn't the negative beliefs themselves that cause us so many issues, but the painful feelings that accompany them. Most people have a certain feeling that always crops up in the foreground, and that could be seen as "their" issue. For some, this might be a feeling of abandonment and loneliness. For others, it's insecurity and shame. Some people suffer inflated feelings of guilt, whereas others are overcome with anxiety. Many are racked with envy, others with lethargy. Countless people are regularly flooded with feelings of depression.

It can be difficult to regulate these feelings or moods, depending on their level of intensity. Brain research has shown that any extreme state of excitation—whether linked to positive or negative feelings—will block access to our knowledge of the fitting solution. That's why the earlier we recognize it's time for our inner adult to intervene, the better. I'd like to use another example from my practice to illustrate.

Suzie, thirty-two, suffers from extreme insecurity and self-doubt. During one session, she told me about how she had spent an entire evening watching her crush dance with someone else. She then spent the rest of the weekend in bed, depressed. Suzie said that once she started feeling this way, there was no escape. Her crush ignoring her and choosing to dance with someone else all night had really eroded her self-esteem, which unleashed the depression. She could have avoided this mental tailspin had she taken care of herself sooner—had she caught herself in time to realize that she was channeling her shadow child, whose beliefs included "It's all my fault" and "I'm a burden." Suzie could have then comforted her shadow child, explaining that who this man chose to dance with had absolutely no bearing on the shadow child's worth. Her inner adult could have shown the shadow child that it was currently experiencing "mirrored self-esteem" (see page 33). Furthermore,

Suzie's inner adult could have pointed out that the shadow child always developed crushes on moody, difficult men (there was a history there), and that this guy certainly wasn't worth ruining their night over. Finally, adult Suzie could have seen to it that she either spent the evening enjoying herself with other people on the dance floor, or she could have left the club and found something else to do. She could have met up with a friend or gone to her favorite bar, where a friendly chat with an old acquaintance would have distracted her and cheered her up. The problem was that yet again, Suzie had failed to realize that she was identifying wholly with her shadow child that night, and had simply endured the pain rather than intervening and taking care of herself.

If you want to regulate or even avoid certain feelings, you must be certain to take care of yourself in time. If your shadow child tends toward feelings of abandonment and loneliness, and you happen to be single currently, then see to it that you avoid things that trigger this feeling. For instance, make sure that you have enough planned for Sundays so you don't fall into that pit of loneliness.

If you're often jealous, then do yourself a favor by preparing a few strategies to help you regulate this feeling. For example, if you and your partner are invited to a party, arm your shadow child against possible situations in which your jealousy might flare up. Think about the ways in which you can keep your adult-self in charge. Identify potential triggers in advance, and keep your behavior strategies at the ready.

We usually slip into painful emotional states because we haven't prepared for difficult situations, and/or because we don't catch it soon enough when the shadow child starts taking the wheel. Some emotional states are easy to regulate, because we know what the triggers are and do our best to avoid them. For instance, if I'm trying to get clean, I'll do whatever it takes not to come into contact with my poison. For most emotional states, though, it makes more sense not to try avoiding the triggers, which often isn't even possible. Instead, we should prepare the strategies we need to manage them. To illustrate this point, I would like to examine individuals whose self-protection strategies are aggression and attack, because these people live with seemingly uncontrollable feelings of rage.

SIDE NOTE: THE IMPULSIVE SHADOW CHILD

Impulsive people exhibit a hair-trigger stimulus-response connection. This means that almost no time elapses between the thing that makes them mad and their reaction to it. Think of Michael from the opening of this book, the guy who lost his mind over his partner forgetting to buy him a bag of chips. He's a typical example of a person with this self-protection strategy.

If you're like Michael, try to identify the actual cause of

your rage. In Michael's case, it only appeared as though the chips were the problem. In actuality, his anger was prompted by his wounded shadow child and its beliefs that "I'm coming up short" and "No one takes my wishes seriously." In other words, Michael's anger is generated by his interpretation of reality. It's especially important for people prone to impulsive, angry outbursts to know what sets them off, because it's here that prevention has to start. Rage has to be caught in its early stages, if not kept from arising, altogether. Once your blood starts to boil, there's no turning back. But if we prepare and get to know our triggers, we're giving our inner adult the best possible chance to respond calmly. If you know that your parents, coworker, or adolescent kids can quickly set you off, you can arm yourself with your inner adult's help, identifying which buttons they push and deciding in advance how you're going to respond. To identify your triggers, repeat the "Reality Check" on page 213. Figure out what the connections are between the objective occurrence and your subjective perspective. The various situations that have enraged you can probably be distilled down to your negative beliefs, or rather, to your shadow child's wounds.

Marcus, thirty-two, had a very difficult childhood. His parents were both violent alcoholics. Considering his childhood, it was amazing how well he was getting by as an adult. The only thing that kept causing him trouble was his impulsivity. His shadow child was very sensitive and would break down whenever Marcus got the feeling he wasn't being shown enough respect. All it would take was (what he read as) a funny look from someone at the bar. Marcus would think he was being provoked, that people were laughing at him. His verbal assault immediately followed, often ending in physical violence. When Marcus made the acquaintance of his shadow child, he identified a litany of negative beliefs. One of the most prominent was "I'm powerless." Feelings of powerlessness and helplessness were the hotbed of his impulsive rage. The same can be said for a lot of people who tend toward aggression and attack. After all, aggression serves the evolutionary purpose of freeing us from this very state.

In order to regulate his anger, Marcus had to learn to take his shadow child lovingly by the hand and stay situated in his adult-self—in other words, on level footing with his suspected antagonists. To accomplish this, he did a lot of the exercises presented in this book. What also really helped was the practice of *response strategies*, which I'll introduce in the section after next. Response strategies reduce the feeling of subjective helplessness and can provide a certain sense of composure. Speaking of composure, it's not only feelings of inferiority that give rise to rage. People in superior positions are also known to allow their aggression free rein. All the time, bosses vent their frustration on subordinates, parents yell at their children, teachers reprimand their students, etc. And unquestionably, people who are on equal footing will also attack one another. Rage builds up whenever things aren't going the way we want. It really doesn't take much more than feeling as though our partner has misunderstood us, or discovering that the dishwasher wasn't emptied. Anger is a reaction to loss of control. Impatience plays a big part in this as well—it could be seen as anger's little sister. Impulsive individuals are usually impatient. But impulsivity isn't just an experience; it isn't natural law or a twist of fate. We have control over our impulsivity, which everyone with this proclivity must admit to themselves. A tiny glimmer of free will precedes every tantrum. This is how a hothead somehow manages to keep it together for their boss, but not—evidently—for their family. Indeed, a client once told me that she was able to tamp down her angry outbursts with the help of a single sentence that had occurred to me (without any sense of its ultimate impact): "Just let it be."

COW MEDITATION

Humor is a great antidote to anger. To that end, I'd like to share a little story: I was at one of my workshops with my friend Helena, who is also a psychotherapist and was helping me lead the workshop. We were sitting together one evening, when out of the clear blue sky, she told me to make a cow face.

I said, "No way!"

"Yes, do it," she insisted.

Well, I managed to hold the stupid face for a few seconds before I burst out laughing. Helena, who practices in East Frisia in northern Germany, then told me that she would sometimes do what she called *cow meditation* with her clients. This wasn't too great a stretch for East Frisians, Helena added, because the region had more cows than people. She would have her client make a cow face, and then mimic them and tell them to get really mad. The client would respond, "I can't," to which she said, "Precisely!" It was impossible to make a cow face and be angry at the same time, Helena explained. Cows have such a relaxed and innocent look that can't be reconciled with rage. Helena thus suggested a daily ten-minute-long cow meditation to those clients who were frequently irritable and grumpy. I would like to second this suggestion.

As a reminder to your inner adult, our posture and facial expression have a direct influence on our mood. A thoroughly relaxed, even bovine, facial expression is physiologically at odds with rage.

* * *

Exercise: A Little Lesson in Quick-Wittedness

If you haven't yet mastered cow meditation to the point that you can blithely let attacks roll off you, then response strategies might help you keep your cool. These are little prepared responses that fit any occasion. In his book *Quick-Wittedness* (not yet translated into English), Matthias Nölke refers to these sentences as *instant quips*, an allusion to instant soup or instant coffee. The sentence is formulated in advance, ready to use when the moment arises—the mental effort required borders on zero. If you had to come up with a clever retort on the spot, meanwhile, the moment would probably pass.

Generally speaking, there are two situations in which we would usually like to have a quick-witted response up our sleeve:

1. Teasing but good-natured banter with friends and colleagues. The digs are harmless and can be brushed off with a laugh.
2. Blatant or passive-aggressive attacks that are much more upsetting or hurtful.

The following instant quips can be used in response to almost any real or suspected taunts:

- Did you just say something?
- Could you repeat that backward?
- When in Rome . . .
- If I wanted to hear your opinion, I'd tell you what it is.
- Look who's talking!
- I guess I'm just a square peg in a round hole.

On Self-Protection and Self-Reflection Strategies

The last response is what Nölke terms a *nonsense quips*. These are retorts that don't actually make any sense and thus pull the rug out from under your attacker. They have to think about it for a minute, before realizing *you're* teasing *them*. The same rule applies to so-called *null quips*. These make no sense in the context of your conversation and redirect the attack into the realm of the absurd. In fact, Nölke also writes about the *theater of the absurd*. Here it's important that you remain serious and, in your expression and voice, appear to respond to what was said, but then say something really odd, like "Farmers harvest asparagus in spring" or "A barber learns to shave by shaving fools." The latter is one of the many meaningless expressions you should keep up your sleeve. You can also adulterate familiar expressions, like saying "A bird in the bush is worth two in the hand." These lines confuse people, thus interrupting the usual downward spiral of attack-counterattack. Ideally, both of you will start laughing.

A good way to defuse the attack and introduce some humor to the situation is to take what was said, then exaggerate it. If you're being accused of doing something stupid, all you have to do is say, "That's not the half of it" or "I'm bad at cooking, too!"

Think of situations that are hard to manage, then take some time to craft instant quips you could pull out at those moments. The knowledge that you'll always have a good response at the ready makes you feel stronger and reduces insecurity.

Incidentally, another really good instant quip is "You're right!" This even works with insults, because it shows your attacker how confident you are. So confident, in fact, that you don't take their abuse seriously.

GO AHEAD—DISAPPOINT PEOPLE

People whose self-protection strategies include remaining a child don't dare take responsibility for their own life decisions. The fear they have of doing something wrong is accompanied by a vague (at best) notion of what they actually want. They spend their whole life adjusting to others, which stunts the development of their autonomous skills, including personal volition. As a result, they have no practice standing on their own two feet. Their shadow child thinks it needs to be held by the hand and guided through life. Their adult-self rarely has a say in matters and needs to be bolstered. The shadow child depends on the approval of its parents and other people. It is desperate to meet everyone's expectations. It's afraid of disappointing people. The solution to which reads: *Go ahead—disappoint them!*

A personal sense of right and wrong is needed to detach from our parents. We need to believe in our ability to make decisions and stick by them. This means taking responsibility for our wrong decisions, too, which requires a certain frustration tolerance, which I described at length in the section "Trust in Yourself and in Life" on page 271. We have to be able to endure failure. It's the price we must pay for free will. If I delegate all my decisions to my parents or partner out of fear of possible failure, I will remain forever dependent.

If this sounds like you, please remind your shadow child that it will survive failure, and that negative feelings always pass. Failure is part of life. Tell your shadow child that it's actually far more likely to experience success along the way. The only true failure would be not trying at all, and thus remaining reliant on others. Take your shadow child onto your lap and explain that it's okay to make mistakes. Mistakes are our best teacher. After all, we require a certain degree of psychological strain to grow. When everything's going along smoothly, there's no reason to think about ourselves and make changes. Make sure your adult-self understands that most decisions can also be reversed. If it turns out a decision you made was wrong, you can change it. "What's the worst that could happen?" is an important question in this case as well. It might help to realize that if you remain stuck in your current situation, you'll endure a lot of negative feelings there, too.

Furthermore, tell your shadow child that it's allowed to be disappointing. Explain that its parents are big and can take care of themselves. It's allowed to detach from them. This doesn't mean you don't love your parents anymore; all it means is that you are now shaping your life the way you want. By the same token, you have every right to detach from your partner, as necessary.

As I wrote in the section "Self-Protection Strategy: I'll Remain a Child" (page 116), some people have parents and/or partners who want to be in charge and can become downright coercive. If this sounds like you, please stop trying to sugarcoat things. Stop denying the gravity of this situation. Do you live in constant hope of your parents or partner changing one day? With the help of your inner adult, soberly take stock of the situation and make a *realistic* prediction of the chances for improvement. Are you unsure whether you might be to blame for your difficulties with this person? Perhaps because they always say you are? If so, assess your own standpoint by means of argumentation. The sections on conflict management starting on page 241 can help.

You don't need to take all these steps at once. What's important is that you start on your path to independence. For example, before breaking abruptly from your partner, practice contradicting them more often and standing up for your point of view. It might also help to start with small decisions that you pledge to make and see through.

SIDE NOTE: SELF-REFLECTION STRATEGIES AGAINST ADDICTION

As we've learned, habitual thoughts and behaviors give rise to neuronal connections that often make us behave in automatic, unconscious ways. In its own right, this automation is pretty useful and economical. Otherwise, everyday activities like brushing our teeth, driving, or talking on the phone would require our full attention and presence of mind. Life would be really draining. The downside to the whole story is that our bad habits also become deeply imprinted upon our brains. And when a habit transforms into necessity, what we're looking at is addiction.

Addiction is a very broad field, and there are many detailed self-help books on different types of addiction and how to overcome them. I would therefore like to limit our focus here to a handful of self-reflection strategies that can help you let go of your dependency.

Addictions have such control over us because they affect our feelings. Using a certain drug or pursuing an addictive behavior can cause feelings of pleasure. It can also prevent strong feelings of pain or discomfort, such as symptoms of withdrawal. Although the sun child can play a part in the former scenario, given its proclivity toward high spirits and excess, the negative feelings of the latter are situated firmly with the shadow child. The idea of going without a certain drug unleashes feelings of fear, at least subliminally. The shadow child fears that without this substance, it will lose its inner support. Oral addictions—such as drinking, smoking, and eating—are closely tied to the shadow child's desire for protection and security. On a deep, unconscious level, oral consumption is tied to the feelings of human affection and being breast-fed. The shadow child needs comforting and affection. Drugs can ease its pain in the short term.

In addition to the shadow child's addictions rooted in desire, dependency can also be influenced by metabolic variables. Some people's dopamine circulatory systems make them more susceptible to addiction than others. Studies also recently discovered that some people break down nicotine quickly, whereas others process it more slowly. The first group is far more likely to become addicted to cigarettes than the second. Addiction is not just the territory of sad shadow children; many factors contribute to it, including opportunity and habit.

It takes a strong will to free ourselves from addiction, which takes a strong inner adult, because free will falls within its purview. This represents a vicious cycle, however, since an addict's will is most often governed by their dependency. The question that emerges is, how can the inner adult regain control over its free will? After all, we experience our free will as something of an event. For instance, we'll wake up one morning and announce, "As of today, no more [overeating, smoking, drinking, putting up with a bad relationship, etc.]." Where did this resolve come from all of a sudden? Why didn't it appear sooner? And even trickier: How long will it last? Many psychological studies have examined this final question and concluded that free will operates as a sort of muscle that can also be exhausted through overexertion. In other words, our willpower weakens the more often we use it. For instance, when we've spent the whole day denying ourselves certain things and delaying gratification, by the time evening rolls around, our willpower has begun to flag. This is why our best intentions tend to fall apart at night, which anyone who has ever been on a diet could tell you.

As I wrote in the special case "Descent Into Addiction" (page 128), dependency is a behavior dictated by its consequences. If the price of continuing greatly exceeds that of quitting, this will then inspire us to stop the behavior. It's here that we can position the lever for change. Addiction requires a considerable level of suppression to function. Although the inner adult knows that its addiction is harmful, it won't admit this knowledge to itself. In other words, your inner adult will suppress the fear you feel at your own behaviors. This comes quite easily, because the health consequences of addiction are typically long-term, meaning you can put off thinking about them. Meanwhile, the short-term enjoyment is immediately felt. The pleasure floods in the moment I light my cigarette or polish off that bar of chocolate. As for the purely theoretical consideration of what long-term effects my behaviors may have, I don't feel a blessed thing.

Central to the overall feelings we experience is the sensation of being alive. In this regard, every addiction can be tied to an existential sensation that the addict loves. The longer an addiction is at play, the more comprehensive the network of neuronal connections built around this feeling. An addicted brain has very little capacity to create neuronal pathways for alternative behaviors. Whereas a massive network of data superhighways exists for addictive behaviors in the brain, other behaviors not associated with the dependency are provided little more than an overgrown neuronal footpath, if anything at all. This is why addicts are often unable even to *imagine* life without their drugs.

Healing an addiction is further complicated by the fact that we're required to *refrain* from a particular behavior. Refraining is a lot tougher than simply doing something, because it's a 24/7 undertaking. Overall, *not* doing something takes far more willpower than doing it. If I decide to go jogging for half an hour a day, all I need is willpower for those thirty minutes, plus five minutes beforehand to get changed. Refraining from doing something, however, takes a whole day's worth of resolve.

If I want to find a way to quit, then, I'll need to position the lever for change in various spots: I have to calm my deeper fears, or rather, comfort my shadow child; change my sensation of being alive with the help of my shadow and sun child; and, as part of that, strengthen the will of my inner adult. The following measures will help expand that footpath into a highway.

1. Dig deep inside yourself to ask your shadow child why it needs this addiction. As explained earlier, addiction has a lot to do with comfort and security—or rather, with

fear. Fear of failure, fear of abandonment, fear of decline and death. Examine which negative beliefs play key roles in your dependency. This will go beyond the ones you've already discovered, such as "I'm not good enough" or "I'm worthless," to include beliefs related directly to your addiction, like "This'll never work," "I can't be happy without smoking," or "I *need* to eat sweets." Get a real sense for how this makes you feel. Identify the negative feeling that pushes you toward drugs. Please write down everything you discover about your shadow child and your addiction.

2. Then take your shadow child onto your lap and comfort it. Explain that you understand its fears, but that they won't go away if you overeat or drink too much, smoke, or bury yourselves in work. Explain that you—the loving inner adult—are there for your shadow child and will never let it down. Tell the child that together, you can do anything. Make sure it knows how proud and happy it will be if and when it manages to quit. Describe how beautiful life will be then.

3. Admit your fear of what could happen if you keep doing what you're doing. Face this reality squarely. Make it very clear to yourself that your behavior *is* harmful. Enter the chamber of horrors that is your fear, and pull up the consequences of your addiction, the horrible images

that you usually suppress. Stop suppressing. Admit to the fears you have. Fear serves the purpose of warning us. In this case, it's justified.

4. Remind yourself that there's always tomorrow, and that by thinking, "I'll quit tomorrow/next week/next year," you can delay your healing till the day you die.

5. Ask your sun child why it loves this addiction. As we know, the sun child is also drawn to play, having fun, partying, and excess. It loves feeling this way. Get a clear sense of how this positive, addictive sensation feels, and where it lives in your body. Identify the positive beliefs associated with your addiction, such as "I'm indestructible," "I'm getting high on *life*," and "I can quit later." Write down everything you discover about your sun child and your addiction.

Search for a new sensation of being alive that satisfies both your shadow child and your sun child. For instance, if you overeat—thus providing your shadow child with feelings of safety and comfort—try to set an entirely new stage in your mind. Picture this: You're living on a tropical island, where all you eat is fruit, vegetables, and fresh fish. Engaging all of your senses, imagine the beautiful sensation created by the warmth, the colors, and the light fare. Picture how it feels to be light and nimble yourself. There is nothing limiting the scope of your imagination here. Create images in your mind that incorporate your new eating habits. Most important, *feel* how good it feels. Mentally immerse yourself in this new sensation. Remember: Our brain doesn't differentiate much between reality and imagination. If you create this gorgeous movie set in your mind, and use it to explore these novel feelings, the first lane of your brain's new data superhighway will be added.

If you want to quit smoking, you could perhaps imagine yourself spending time in a beautiful forest, really connecting with the landscape. Breathing in the fresh air. It's also nice to imagine swimming vigorously in the ocean, then lying on the beach, out of breath, and soaking in the warmth of the sun to recharge. You're so out of breath that smoking would be completely out of the question. Imagine how much cleaner and nicer it would be if you no longer had to walk around with a cigarette between your lips. Smell the pleasant aroma that will surround you when you no longer smoke.

Or create a different inner place to visit whenever you need to experience feelings of peace and deep relaxation. These images calm your shadow child's fear and fulfill your sun child's desires.

6. Develop helpful new beliefs that correspond to this new sensation of being alive and weave them into the images you're seeing. Get a good sense of how these statements feel in your body. Write them out in your favorite color

on a piece of paper, and hang it up at home. Recite these lines at least fifteen times a day, and really *feel* them.

7. Like I said, it's very hard *not* to do something, so come up with something to do *instead*. Create a counter-regimen that extends beyond your imagination to your actual behaviors. Exercise is one of the best "drugs" to combat addiction, and it can lead you to an entirely new way of life. If you don't already, I highly recommend you start exercising regularly.

    Think of all the great things you can do to fill the supposed void caused by quitting drugs. Maybe you'll pick up a new hobby, seek out professional retraining, or take a class. Do whatever feels good and gives your life joy and meaning. And be sure to plan rewards for yourself at different milestones of addiction-free living.

8. Whenever a craving sets in, turn to this new sensation of being alive and allow yourself to be distracted by it. Whatever you do, don't get caught up in the craving—distraction is the name of the game. It practically goes without saying, but, as best you can, try to avoid temptation.

Furthermore, daily structure can be very helpful in preventing cravings from arising in the first place. Most relapses occur when we're under a lot of stress or have too much time on our hands. Structure can help me avoid both. More on that in the next section.

SHAKE OFF YOUR LETHARGY

Lethargy, or sluggishness, is one of our biggest obstacles when we're trying to reshape our lives and usher in change. Like so many human traits, lethargy also has a genetic component: In addition to an internal "active" setting, our bodies can also switch into "power-save mode." This allowed our ancestors to conserve their energy, so they wouldn't needlessly wear themselves out. Lethargy and laziness are as innate to humans as activity and ambition. You've probably experienced it yourself that the more you relax, the more lethargic you become, and the more you do, the more energy you have. Both states are self-reinforcing. This is reflected in the law of inertia, which states that an object at rest stays at rest unless acted upon by an external force, and a body in motion stays in motion unless acted upon by an external force that changes its direction or speed.

I had a crazy experience with this when I was a student: Summer vacation had finally started, which I'd been looking forward to for ages. My to-do list was a mile long, and now that exams were over, I finally had time to take care of it. The first three weeks of vacation were spent doing a bunch of different things. By then, I'd pretty much worked my way through the list. Suddenly I had all this free time. Too much free time. Because there wasn't any real reason to get up in the morning, I'd bring my coffee back to bed with me and spend hours reading. My blood never had a chance to get flowing. Toward noon, because I hadn't moved, I was tired enough to fall back asleep. By the time I woke up later in the afternoon, my system had completely bottomed out. I felt terrible, drank more coffee, and tried to pull myself together and—if I was lucky—get a little done around the apartment. In the evening, I looked back on my utterly unproductive day. It made me unhappy. I was pretty good at suppressing this unhappiness at night, though, when I would go to house parties or hit the bars. The less I had to do, the lazier I became. My level of inactivity was so extreme that by the end of summer vacation, it was all I could do to run a load of laundry on days that were otherwise completely open. I was delighted when school started and my days had structure again. I was instantly back up to speed and could suddenly manage three loads of laundry on top of my hefty workload, and all without a single complaint.

And that's not just me. Lots of people need external pressures and a set daily structure, in order to operate. It's easiest for us to remain active when we don't lose speed in the first place. Mondays aren't the worst day of the week because demands on us are any higher—it's because the contrast to the weekend is so stark. It takes much more *motivation* to survive Monday than Tuesday. Work feels even easier on Wednesday, and by Friday, we can't remember why we felt so crummy at the start of the week. It's the same with any other activity that takes a certain level of determination and effort. The more we do these activities, the easier they come.

Clear structure to your day is thus the best prevention against lethargy. Map out your daily and weekly schedule, including free time activities. I adhere pretty strictly to the schedules I set for myself, and as a result, I have more free time than most people. I exercise a little before breakfast. I spend my morning writing. During the lunch hour, I'll hang out some, then practice piano. I work as a psychotherapist in the afternoon. My workday ends at six p.m. It might be conventional, but it works. It's the result of the experiences I had as a student. Carefully consider what you want and what's important to you, and build your daily and weekly schedules around it. Schedules—just like to-do lists—are incredibly helpful for getting things done. And they protect you from becoming overwhelmed, which is as detrimental as being underchallenged. People who are bad at managing their time are often stressed out and overwhelmed. They get a lot done at the last minute, which makes them feel constantly harried and under pressure.

Set structures are so important to us because they obviate our need to make new decisions constantly. Our free will and decision-making capacity are closely bound, and both can flag when overtaxed. This has been proven in a range of psychological experiments. One of these experiments tested the decision-making behaviors of German drivers, who were asked to select features for their new car on a computer. Color, interior fittings, engine details—the more decisions the buyers had to make, the more overwhelmed they became and likely to fall back on the base model, despite the fact that this cost about 1,500 euros more on average. When you have a defined schedule, only *one* decision remains for you to make, namely whether you'll stick to it. Of course there will be exceptions. I'm not exactly as stringent as I made myself out to be above. But given the fact that the metaplan exists, I always find my way back to my beneficial routines.

The biggest problem is usually just getting started. This can require a lot of motivation. It's a lot easier after the fact, especially if I stick to it and do it regularly. After all, if you don't use it, you lose it. This even applies to sex—at least in established relationships, where the passion may have waned.

Speaking of passion: This could be considered the alternative to discipline. I don't know a single person whose work is powered by passion alone. Even artists will usually follow strict working hours. Every activity or acquisition of skills will go through the occasional dry spell. It takes stamina to get through these periods. People who lack stamina will start a lot of things, but see very little through. Their expertise and knowledge will thus remain superficial. They don't dig deeper into the material. This makes them unhappy over time. They don't have anything that they really throw themselves into. Dedication to a task or activity, digging deeper and deeper over time, can give us profound pleasure and a sense of fulfillment. It boosts our self-esteem in a healthy way. I'll go into this more in the section "Pursue Your Hobbies and Interests" on page 307.

If I'm trying to shake off my lethargy, it's also important to look at how to boost my motivation and stamina. This applies in particular to chronic procrastinators, who constantly put off critical tasks. Procrastinators usually suffer not only the effects of their power-save mode, but also their shadow child's pronounced self-doubt. A procrastinator's shadow child is usually afflicted with fear of failure. Their subliminal fear of not being up to a certain task—of simply not being able to do it—makes them put it off. As is so often the case, their inner adult may see things differently. Of course the inner adult knows that they can successfully do their taxes or clean up the basement, but the shadow child—with its vague fears of failure—prevails. Its beliefs might include "I can't do it," "I'm too weak," or "I'm so dumb." Procrastination is thus a special manifestation of the flight and avoidance self-protection strategy. If the shadow child isn't party to the procrastination, though, then the individual has simply fallen victim to lethargy. The tips I share in the next section can help.

Sometimes, however, the procrastinator's shadow child can also be petulant. In such cases, the shadow child has a hard time dealing with other people's expectations. People who are caught up in the autonomy-dependence conflict (see page 28) will often refuse requests, because they see them as limiting their personal freedom. In other words, they take the one thing that's expected of them—and they don't do it. Passive aggression is often the self-protection strategy hiding behind procrastination. More on that in the section "Break Down Your Resistance" on page 304. First, I'd like to give you a few tips for combatting procrastination.

* * *

Exercise: Seven Steps Against Procrastination

1. Ask your shadow child why it has such a hard time starting things. Is it afraid of failure? Is it being a brat by defying expectations, or is it simply too lazy? Identify the beliefs blocking your way, such as "You can kiss my ass" or "I can't do it." Then try to imagine how it will feel if you keep yielding to this obstinacy or whatever it is that's crippling you. How will you feel this evening, tomorrow, next week, or next month if you keep putting things off? You'll probably experience deep guilt, and maybe even fear. Allow yourself to feel these things.

2. Make a clear distinction between the shadow child and adult within you, and work with both, as you've learned to do in this book. For instance, you can comfort your inner child, bolster the adult with arguments, dismantle your projections, and so on.

3. Reformulate your negative beliefs as positive statements, like you learned to do in "Discover Your Positive
   Beliefs" on page 180. For instance, if you believe "I can't
   do it," then transform this statement into "I can do it." If
   you haven't already, write these positive beliefs down in
   your favorite color, either on the picture of your sun child
   (see page 180) or on a new piece of paper.

4. Feel your goal: If you've been putting off a task with a
   clear deadline, such as filing your taxes, then engage all
   your senses to imagine how it will feel once you've accomplished the task. Or if you're avoiding starting a regular activity—such as exercise—tap into exactly how it
   will feel when you're well into an established exercise
   routine and those painful first workout sessions have
   faded into the past. Fully embrace this positive feeling—
   activate your sun child.

5. Set intermediate goals if the task appears insurmountable. For example, if you want to start jogging, begin by
   spending half an hour switching between walking and
   running. This isn't as challenging and thus reduces that
   initial hurdle. If you want to clean the basement, you
   don't need to squander an entire week of vacation on the
   task. If you think that way, you may never turn your intention into action. Instead, set yourself the goal of taking
   just an hour every evening to clean. In short: Create realistic, easily actionable objectives.

6. Incorporate your plan into your daily and/or weekly schedule.

7. Plan personal rewards: If you managed to work on the basement for an hour every evening for a week, for instance, then treat yourself to something nice. Or ask someone else to treat you. If you did all that hard work while your partner was spared, you could ask them to reward you with a back massage.

Always remember that putting things off can rob you of twenty-four hours a day and seven days a week. The I-can-get-this-behind-me attitude, meanwhile, requires far less time and effort.

BREAK DOWN YOUR RESISTANCE

There are countless people whose inner child is trapped by its own defiance. I've already written at some length about people whose shadow child demonstrates an exaggerated craving for autonomy in the sections "Autonomy and Dependence in Conflict" on page 28 and "Self-Protection Strategy: The Power Hungry" on page 107. Their behavior is usually in response to the excessive control their parents wielded in their childhood. Their shadow child got stuck in its defiant phase. They reflexively resist any expectations other people have of them. In order to prove their autonomy, they do the very opposite of what's expected of them. They're effectively boycotting not only their relationships, but, first and foremost, themselves. By refusing to meet any of the demands or expectations of their environment, these individuals end up taking a lot of needless detours and breaks. In their professional life, it isn't uncommon for these people to perform far below their potential, because their shadow child mulishly insists on defying their parents' expectations. Many are also commitment-phobes, because the intimacy of a close relationship is too great a threat to their need for autonomy. Relationships feel like prison to them, and they fear for their personal freedom. The shadow child within them believes that it *must* submit to their partner's expectations in order to be loved, and this closeness can rapidly make them feel as though they've lost themselves. For that reason, they will often reestablish distance after close personal moments. They require solitude to feel truly in touch with themselves.

If this is hitting close to home, keep reminding your shadow child that you're big now, and all grown up. You don't need to constantly prove to yourself that you have power, by refusing certain things. Analyze your defiance based on concrete situations in which it always emerges. Suss out the beliefs underlying this behavior. Common ones include "I'm responsible for your happiness," "I always have to be there for you," "I have to adjust," "I'm not allowed to defend myself," and "I can't just be me." Your shadow child compensates for these beliefs by exercising active and passive resistance toward them. With the help of your inner adult, make it crystal clear that as a slave to these behaviors, you lack as much autonomy as you would meeting people's expectations of you. After all, when you always have to know what someone else wants, so you can then decide what you *don't* want, it doesn't exactly make you the stronger one in the equation.

Your problem is that you have a hard time disengaging from other people's expectations, and as a result, you don't actually know what you want. Because you struggle to assert yourself, you isolate yourself that much more radically from other people's expectations, whether real or invented in your mind. In other words, you try to escape by getting out in front of things. If you want to break this pattern, it's very important that your shadow child understand that you're a free human being and grown up now. Your shadow child is caught in the reality of the past, when Mommy and Daddy still had all the say.

Before you're able to make any truly autonomous decisions about what you do and don't want, you have to feel—deep down inside—that you are a free person now. Then you can feel good about saying yes, because you'll know that *you* are the one who made the call, and you'll no longer feel governed by other people's expectations. It's very important that first, you establish a better connection to your desires and needs, and second, you learn to assert yourself in an appropriate manner so you don't get stuck putting up stubborn resistance again.

When interacting with people, keep a close eye on how you're feeling and what you would like to say or do. In these moments, pay especially close attention to whether your instinct is to please the people you're with. This is the reason for your resistance, after all. Your shadow child is perpetually afraid of slipping into an inferior stance. This is why it demands so much freedom, independence, and, thus, power. Whenever you start feeling defiant, summon your adult-self and analyze the situation with a clear mind. It's all about constantly reminding yourself that you are on equal footing with the people around you. You have the same rights, and you are free. Then evaluate whether it's fair and right for you to boycott this person's wishes. You're usually so concerned with protecting your own boundaries that you lose all sense of empathy for others. When you're channeling your defiant shadow child, whoever you're with can quickly mutate into an adversary. Question and correct your perception as often as possible. There are lots of exercises in this book that can help.

PURSUE YOUR HOBBIES AND INTERESTS

Work and activity make us happy, whereas lethargy brings us down—Thomas Aquinas made this case a long time ago. Activity serves as an antidepressant and can allow us to forget ourselves, which is a huge relief to our emotional life. These are the findings of extensive studies on the feeling of happiness. A pioneer in this field was the psychologist Mihály Csíkszent-mihályi, who developed the notion of *flow*. Flow refers to an inner state in which a person becomes completely absorbed in whatever they're doing. In flow, I forget myself. I can enter this state while gardening, skiing, working on crafts, making music—any activity I really throw myself into. Dedication to an activity pushes our skills and gives us the feeling we're doing something meaningful. It sends us straight to our sun child state.

If you don't have many outside interests or hobbies, I highly recommend you expand this area of your life. Think about what would make you happy, and start there. Never think you're too old for something. There are lots of things we pick up quickly as adults because we have better learning strategies than children. For instance, contrary to popular belief, adults learn to play instruments with greater ease than kids do. I didn't start playing the piano till age forty-two, and I made rapid progress.

Hobbies and outside interests help redirect your attention to things beyond yourself. They distract you from self-centered concerns. And the happiness and pride you feel at improving or learning something new is truly wonderful. It's a healthy way to boost your self-esteem. It calms your shadow child and delights your sun child when you dedicate your focus and enthusiasm to an activity.

Hobbies and interests help you discover your own fulfillment. Cultivating your interests is entirely up to you. You don't need to wait around for someone else to make you happy or to do something that makes you feel better. As you gain new skills, keep in mind that there will always be dry spells along the way. If you're one of those people who starts a lot but finishes very little, spend some more time with the section "Shake Off Your Lethargy" on page 297.

By pursuing your hobbies and interests, you are taking responsibility for your own well-being. This naturally also applies to activities that we don't do regularly, such as having friends over for dinner, going to the movies, or hitting the public pool in summer. Don't wait around for something to happen—shape every part of your life.

That was just an overview of the most important self-reflection strategies. You may have been doing some of them for years already, while others were less familiar. As we've discussed, it all comes down to how we shape our relationships. The better our relationship with ourselves, the happier our relationships with others. The closer an eye I keep on my shadow child, the less likely I am to project my fears and shortcomings onto other people, and the less I fall back on my self-protection strategies, which tend to harm my relationships more than they help. The more often I channel my sun child, the easier time I have showing goodwill toward myself and others.

As I described in "The Four Basic Psychological Needs" on page 25, everything in life centers around just a handful of things: connection versus self-assertion, control versus trust, along with pleasure, displeasure, and self-esteem. That said, I would argue that self-esteem is the foundation for it all. It's what determines how well I can balance my needs for connection on the one hand and self-assertion on the other. It also determines the level of control I require in order to feel safe or able to trust. Self-esteem even influences our need to feel pleasure and avoid displeasure; a person with strong self-esteem is far better able to regulate these needs than someone who is deeply insecure. They don't have the need for compulsive discipline, nor do they succumb to exorbitant self-indulgence.

The shadow child and the sun child are metaphors for our self-esteem, which has its weak, problematic areas as well as its strong, healthy parts. As you are now well aware, it all comes down to accepting your shadow child, without allowing it to take the reins. That, and bolstering your sun child and giving it much more space in your life. The things that weigh on each of our minds are, of course, highly individualized, which is why I designed the introduction to the shadow child and the sun child in such a way that each reader could fill in their own personal details. The next step is to take note of the self-reflection strategies that are most important to you, and that you would like to start seeing and developing in your everyday life.

* * *

Exercise: Find Your Personal Self-Reflection Strategies

Of the self-reflection strategies introduced earlier, please se-lect the ones you feel would be especially helpful to you. As with the self-protection strategies, you may certainly add self-reflection strategies that I failed to mention explicitly, or you can formulate your own that are highly specific to you. For in-stance, you may write down, "I'm learning saxophone," "I main-tain equal footing with my husband," "I start every day by engaging my sun child feeling," "I'm looking for a new job," or "I play with my (real) kids for half an hour every day." Add your personal self-reflection strategies to the feet of your sun child drawing (see image inside the front cover).

You now have your sun child, with all its potential, at your disposal. This potential can only be realized, however, if you regularly *play* with your sun child and *live out* your new beliefs, values, and self-reflection strategies—this means using your new knowledge in everyday life. It means *catching yourself* whenever you start slipping back toward your shadow child. It means *separating* your shadow child from your adult-self and exercising a *calming influence* over your shadow child. It means deliberately *switching over* to your sun child or inner adult as often as possible—which in turn means repeatedly *reminding yourself* of your new beliefs. Think of your values and *implement them* whenever you can. And *practice* your self-reflection strategies. Most important, really *spend time* with the exercises I have introduced here, and keep coming back to them. Accept *responsibility* for your personal development.

To help remind yourself of your newfound knowledge in everyday life, I recommend hanging your sun child drawing somewhere in your home—don't hide it away in a drawer. Take a picture of it with your phone as well, so you always have it close at hand when you're out and about.

* * *

Exercise: Integrating the Shadow Child and the Sun Child

This exercise is intended to help you connect your shadow child and your sun child and integrate them into your personality. The Infinity Walk, in which an individual walks in a figure-eight pattern, was developed by American psychologist and researcher Deborah Sunbeck. Used as a method for developing increasingly complex neuronal networks, the exercise promotes collaboration between the two halves of the brain. For the next exercise, my colleague and friend Julia Tomuschat modified the original Infinity Walk to enable a kinesthetic integration of the states of mind we now know as the shadow child and the sun child. I regularly run this exercise at my workshops and am always impressed by its impact. The objective is to accept and integrate the shadow child and sun child into yourself, and to come away with the clear sense that you have a *choice* between these two states of mind.

It's best to have two helpers for this exercise, but you can also do it alone.

1. Referring to your shadow child drawing (see page 64), write down your negative core beliefs and feelings on a note card or piece of paper. If you'd like, you can add a corresponding color, which in this case could be gray. You could also choose a word like "gloomy," or another atmospheric term that applies to light and darkness. We associate a lot with colors and light, and including this modality here can help.

   Bearing this in mind, on a second note card, write down your positive core beliefs, your feelings, a color, the cue for your inner image (such as "ocean"), and your sun child's values.

2. Place your shadow and sun child note cards on the floor in such a way that you can walk around them in a figure eight. In other words, your shadow child will be inside

one of the (imagined) loops of the eight, your sun child in the other.

3. If you have two helpers, they should position themselves at opposite bends of the eight. Helper A holds the note card representing your shadow child, Helper B that of the sun child.

4. Start from the middle of your imagined eight and begin tracing its outline. Whenever you enter the first loop, Helper A—who is standing on this side—reads from their card. As soon as you reach the junction of the two loops in the middle and start walking into the second loop, Helper B will start reading from the other note card. As soon as you pass through the center, Helper A will start up again, and so on. If you don't have any helpers, just switch off between reading out loud from the two cards. Or make a recording of both cards that you repeat about ten times. It's important that the recording tempo correspond to your walking pace around the figure eight, so that the transitions between cards align with your transitions from one loop into the other.

5. Walk around the figure eight about ten times while you or your helpers read the cards out loud. At the end, stop in the middle of the figure eight and sense what's changed inside you and which state you feel more drawn toward. If you feel drawn toward your shadow child more

than toward your sun child, repeat the exercise as many times as it takes for things to feel good and harmonious.

You can tailor this exercise to all sorts of concerns in your life. It's particularly helpful in reaching a decision when you're feeling conflicted about two contradictory needs or motivations. Write the pros on one note card, cons on the other. If you'd like to get more out of the Infinity Walk, I recommend you read the book by the same name.

We are now approaching the final section of this book. This will also highlight a self-reflection strategy, but one that is so fundamental and all-encompassing that it could easily be considered the ultimate goal of this book, which is why I've saved it for last.

LET YOURSELF *BE* YOURSELF

As I have repeatedly emphasized, we employ self-protection strategies to protect ourselves from attack and to gain as much recognition as possible. Remember, this isn't the result of childhood influences alone, but is also tied to genetic programming: we depend upon connection to a community. Using guilt as leverage, our genes compel us to behave in such a way that allows us to survive socially. Feelings of shame have served the evolutionary purpose of making us adjust to our communities.

Deep humiliation can be downright traumatizing. Shame is an extremely powerful, debilitating feeling. The range of things that we find embarrassing, however, varies significantly between individuals. People whose shadow child exhibits a lot of negative, self-deprecating beliefs are much quicker to feel embarrassed than those who exhibit largely positive beliefs. Many people are ashamed of their personal insecurity. It's not even bad to be insecure, though—everyone is at some point, depending on situation and circumstance. It's fine. It's human.

What's not fine is if I compensate for my feelings of inferiority by concealing my opinions and desires, being aggressive, giving people the runaround, fleeing my relationships, or denigrating other folks.

If we want to start believing in ourselves—as the prerequisite for both our personal freedom and successful relationships—then we must come to accept our own fallibility. We must accept that we make mistakes, have weaknesses, and are vulnerable. If we think we have to be perfect and bulletproof in order to approach life, countless chances and relationships will pass us by.

It doesn't matter if you're good-looking, perfect, and powerful. What matters is that you find yourself. The more loving and safe a home your shadow child and your sun child can find within you, the more peace you'll find, and the better your ability to open up to others with understanding and goodwill. Because home is where you can be *you*. Home means familiarity, security, and stability. Home means belonging. If I become my own home, then I'll belong—connected to myself and others. And that's what it all comes down to in this life.

As the "great philosopher" Popeye always said, "I yam what I yam an' tha's all I yam!" This could become your daily mantra. Self-acceptance doesn't mean that we stop developing, though. On the contrary: I can only work on my shortcomings once I've acknowledged them. Your optimization work should not focus on boosting self-protection strategies, but should instead center on personal behaviors that benefit both you and others. So be happy and proud of yourself whenever

- you muster understanding for your shadow child;
- you stand up for yourself, despite your fear;
- you stand up for someone else, despite your fear;
- you differentiate between fact and interpretation;
- you dismantle your projections;
- you stand by your own arguments, as long as no one has presented any that are better;
- you admit the other person is right, when they're right;
- you handle conflict in an open, fair manner;
- you stand up for your convictions and values;
- you accept responsibility for your feelings and behavior;
- you show generosity toward a difficult person;
- you manage to dismantle feelings of envy;
- you really listen to another person speak;

- you accept a challenge you would have avoided in the past;
- you enjoy your life;
- you're open and honest;
- you live your values;
- you do your exercises every day;
- you sincerely try;
- you live as your sun child.

You are what you are, and that's all that you are,
and what you are is good!

References

Branden, N. (1995). *The Six Pillars of Self-Esteem: The Definitive Work on Self-Esteem by the Leading Pioneer in the Field.* Bantam Books.

Corssen, J. and Tramitz, C. (2014). Ich und die anderen. Als Selbst-Entwickler zu gelingenden Beziehungen. Munich, Knaur.

Dahm, U. (2011). Mit der Kindheit Frieden schließen. Wie alte Wunden heilen. Darmstadt, Schirner.

Dwoskin, H. (2015). *The Sedona Method: Your Key to Lasting Happiness, Success, Peace and Emotional Well-Being.* Sedona Press.

Frankl, V.E. (2006). *Man's Search for Meaning.* Beacon Press.

Gendlin, E. T. (1981). *Focusing.* Bantam Books.

Grawe, Klaus. (2006). *Neuropsychotherapy.* Routledge Press.

Heyman, G. M. (2010). *Addiction: A Disorder of Choice.* Harvard University Press.

Jacob, G. and Arntz, A. (2014). Schematherapie. Fortschritte der Psychotherapie. Göttingen, Hogrefe.

Klein, S. (2005). Einfach glücklich. Die Glücksformel für jeden Tag. Reinbek, Rowohlt.

References

Klein, S. (2010). Der Sinn des Gebens. Warum Selbstlosigkeit in der Evolution siegt und wir mit Egoismus nicht weiterkommen. Frankfurt am Main, Fischer.

Nölke, M. (2009). Schlagfertigkeit. Munich, Haufe.

Reddemann, L. (2002). Imagination als heilsame Kraft. Zur Behandlung von Traumafolgen mit ressourcenorientierten Verfahren. Stuttgart, Klett-Cotta.

Röhr, H.-P. (2013). Die Kunst, sich wertzuschätzen. Angst und Depression überwinden. Selbstsicherheit gewinnen. Ostfildern, Patmos.

Schnarch, D. (2011). *Intimacy and Desire: Awaken the Passion in Your Relationship.* Beaufort Books.

Stahl, S. (2011). Leben kann auch einfach sein! So stärken Sie Ihr Selbstwertgefühl. Hamburg, Ellert & Richter.

Stahl, S. (2014). Jein! Bindungsängste erkennen und bewältigen. Hilfe für Betroffene und deren Partner. Hamburg, Ellert & Richter.

Stahl, S. and Alt, M. (2013). So bin ich eben! Erkenne dich selbst und andere. Hamburg, Ellert & Richter.

Süfke, B. (2010). Männerseelen. Ein psychologischer Ratgeber. Munich, Goldmann.

Sunbeck, D. and Lippmann, E. (2005). Was die 8 möglich macht: Laufend neue Aufgaben lösen. Kirchzarten, VAK.

Unger, H.-P. and Kleinschmidt, C. (2014). "Das hält keiner bis zur Rente durch!" Munich, Kösel.

Index

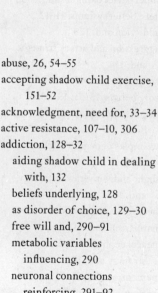

Index

Index